HEART-HEALTHY COOKING FOR ALL SEASONS

HEART-HEALTHY COOKING FOR ALL SEASONS

Conceived by Shep Gordon, Alive Culinary Resources

MARVIN MOSER, M.D.
with
LARRY FORGIONE, JIMMY SCHMIDT,
and ALICE WATERS

POCKET BOOKS

New York   London   Toronto   Sydney   Tokyo   Singapore

POCKET BOOKS, a division of Simon & Schuster Inc.
1230 Avenue of the Americas, New York, NY 10020

Copyright © 1996 by Marvin Moser, M.D., Alive Culinary Resources, Inc., Alice Waters, Larry Forgione, and Jimmy Schmidt
Interior illustrations copyright © 1996 by Lori Almeida

Heart-healthy cooking for all seasons / by Marvin Moser, with Larry
    Forgione, Jimmy Schmidt, and Alice Waters.
        p.   cm.
    Includes index.
    ISBN 0-671-88520-0
    1. Heart—Diseases—Diet therapy.   2. Heart—Diseases—Diet
therapy—Recipes.   3. Heart—Diseases—Prevention.   4. Nutrition.
I. Moser, Marvin, 1924–
RC684.D5H44   1996
641.5'6311—dc20   95-25201
                                                      CIP

First Pocket Books hardcover printing February 1996

10 9 8 7 6 5 4 3 2 1

Interior design by Barbara Scott-Goodman

Printed in the U.S.A.

Acknowledgments

———◦○◦———

We are grateful to Shep Gordon, whose ideas have come to fruition in *Heart-Healthy Cooking for All Seasons*. We are also grateful to Julie Rubenstein of Pocket Books for her helpful suggestions and encouragement. And to Ellen Liskov, a registered dietitian at the Yale–New Haven Hospital, for her meticulous analysis of the recipes. Her advice has been more than helpful in putting together *Heart-Healthy Cooking for All Seasons*. Mary Goodbody, a recognized food writer, was extremely helpful in working with the chefs and putting all of the recipes in good order. Finally, to my wife, Joy, an excellent cook in her own right, for her critique of the manuscript and recipes, as well as her suggestions for the book title.

A brief comment: Physicians learn very little about nutrition, eating habits, obesity, or preventive medicine in medical school. I have learned over the past forty-plus years from experience in counseling people with risk factors for heart disease that there is no easy answer to the question of how to maintain desirable weight and enjoy a nutritious and healthful pattern of eating. But I have also learned that a quick fix and complicated programs don't work. Above all, I have learned that the entrepreneurs of medicine and nutrition are ever present with a new program, a new diet, or a miracle plan. The *science* of good health has not, however, demonstrated that these radical and often difficult-to-follow programs are necessary; changes in behavior that can be accomplished within the framework of one's daily routine will accomplish just as much as rigid programs and not reduce your enjoyment of life. This is why we are convinced that the message of *Heart-Healthy Cooking for All Seasons* is an important one.

Contents

———⊷✦⊶———

FOREWORD   xiii

INTRODUCTION   1

ABOUT WEIGHT   7

CHOLESTEROL: THE MYTHS AND THE FACTS   25

HEART DISEASE AND "HARDENING OF THE ARTERIES"   39

ABOUT THE CHEFS AND THE RECIPES   45

SPRING RECIPES   51

Breakfast
Alice Waters · Compote of Tangerines and Blood Oranges   53
Jimmy Schmidt · Ragout of Citrus with Maple Sugar Crisps   54
Larry Forgione · Fresh Herb and Spinach Omelet   55

Lunch and Salads
Larry Forgione · Jicama, Pineapple, and Watercress Salad   56
Larry Forgione · Poached Oysters and Shrimp with Lemon-Pepper Dressing   57
Larry Forgione · Baked Halibut Fillets with Tomatoes, Capers, and Fresh Herbs   58
Alice Waters · Spring Greens and Radish Salad   59
Alice Waters · Pasta with Bitter Spring Greens   60
Jimmy Schmidt · Radicchio, Watercress, Radish, and Walnut Salad   61
Jimmy Schmidt · Shrimp and Sorrel Risotto   62
Jimmy Schmidt · Ragout of Baby Artichokes and Stuffed Morel Mushrooms   63

Appetizers
Larry Forgione · Chilled Oysters with a Cucumber-Mint Sauce   64
Jimmy Schmidt · Grilled Asparagus with Chervil and Hazelnuts   65
Alice Waters · Grilled Young Leeks on Toast   66

Dinner

Jimmy Schmidt · Halibut, Sweet Pea, and Fines Herbes Stew 67

Jimmy Schmidt · Chicken Grilled with Citrus, Roasted Garlic, and Artichokes 68

Jimmy Schmidt · Rack of Lamb with Jerusalem Artichokes and Mint 70

Alice Waters · Baked Salmon with Watercress Sauce 71

Alice Waters · Spring Turnip Soup 72

Larry Forgione · Grilled Chicken, Forest Mushrooms, and Red Onion Pasta 73

Larry Forgione · Pasta with Grilled Salmon and Garlic Broccoli 74

Larry Forgione · Game Hens with Country Ham and Greens Stuffing and
Bourbon Glaze 75

Dessert

Larry Forgione · Chocolate Cherry Fudge Cake 76

Alice Waters · Strawberry Granita 77

Jimmy Schmidt · Low-Fat Chocolate Brownies 78

SUMMER RECIPES 79

Breakfast

Alice Waters · Millet Muffins with Fresh Corn 81

Jimmy Schmidt · Summer Berry and Maple Pancakes 82

Larry Forgione · Summer Vegetable Frittata 84

Lunch and Salads

Jimmy Schmidt · Sliced Tomatoes, Grilled Onion, and Fried Basil 86

Jimmy Schmidt · Sea Scallops, Red Peppers, and Marjoram Angel Hair Pasta 87

Jimmy Schmidt · Sweet Pepper, Eggplant, Tomato, and Arugula Sandwich 88

Alice Waters · Tomato Confit on Toasted Bread with Pesto 89

Alice Waters · Grilled Vegetable Pasta 91

Alice Waters · Little Multicolored Pepper Pizzas 92

Larry Forgione · Black Bean Salad with Grilled Chicken 94

Larry Forgione · Marinated Seafood Salad with Asparagus 95

Larry Forgione · Grilled New Potato and Artichoke Salad 96

Appetizers

Alice Waters · Rocket Salad with Baked Ricotta 98

Jimmy Schmidt · Spicy Shrimp with Bitter Greens Salad 99

Larry Forgione · Grilled Soft-Shell Crabs and Sweet Potato Salad 100

Dinner

Larry Forgione · Swordfish with Charred Tomato Vinaigrette 101

Larry Forgione · Grilled Veal Chops with Summer Garden Salad 103

Larry Forgione · Herb-Seared Snapper Fillet with Marinated Cucumber
and Tomatoes 104

Larry Forgione · Braised Mahimahi with Fresh Succotash 105

Alice Waters · Summer Minestrone 106

Alice Waters · Baked Salmon 107

Alice Waters · Roast Chicken with Roasted Whole Garlic   108
Jimmy Schmidt · Barbecued Salmon with Roasted Pepper, Sweet Onion,
   and Caper Salsa   109
Jimmy Schmidt · Grilled Breast of Chicken with Sweet Corn and
   Wild Mushroom Salsa   110
Jimmy Schmidt · Chile-Rubbed Tuna with Tomatillo Chutney   112

Dessert
Alice Waters · Compote of White Peaches and Nectarines   113
Alice Waters · Apricot Soufflé   113
Larry Forgione · Angel Food Cake   114
Larry Forgione · Lemon Angel Food Chiffon   115
Jimmy Schmidt · Nectarine and Blackberry Crisp   117

AUTUMN RECIPES   119

Breakfast
Larry Forgione · Warm Apple and Blueberry Compote with Granola and Yogurt   121
Jimmy Schmidt · Apple and Pineapple Muffins   122
Alice Waters · Buckwheat Crepes with Fruit Compote   123

Lunch and Salads
Larry Forgione · Native Bean Soup   124
Larry Forgione · Roasted Corn and Chanterelle Salad with Autumn Greens   125
Larry Forgione · Prosciutto with a Roasted Beet and Fig Salad and a
   Citrus Dressing   127
Alice Waters · Baked Chanterelles with Garlic Toasts   128
Alice Waters · Endive, Apple, and Walnut Salad   129
Alice Waters · Provençal Chicken Salad   130
Jimmy Schmidt · Pork Chops with Mustard and Rosemary   131
Jimmy Schmidt · Spinach, Roasted Pepper, Onion, and Mâche Salad   132
Jimmy Schmidt · Lobster and Quinoa Risotto   133

Appetizers
Larry Forgione · Munchkin Pumpkin with Chanterelles and Lobster in a
   Light Curry Broth   134
Jimmy Schmidt · Grilled Wild Mushrooms with Parsley and Garlic Vinaigrette   136
Alice Waters · Marinated Sardine Fillets   137

Dinner
Alice Waters · Grilled Steak with Gremolata   138
Alice Waters · Pasta with Clams, Thyme, and Garlic   139
Alice Waters · Onion and Roasted Pepper Panade   140
Jimmy Schmidt · Breast of Pheasant or Chicken with Pumpkin and Cranberries   141
Jimmy Schmidt · Duck with Dried Cherries and Sage, Mashed Parsnips
   and Potatoes   142

Jimmy Schmidt · Grilled Salmon with Apples and Juniper 144
Larry Forgione · Roast Chicken with Apple-Sage Dressing 145
Larry Forgione · Venison Pot Roast with Root Vegetables and Parsnip
Whipped Potatoes 148
Larry Forgione · Spicy Grilled Chicken with Apples and Chiles 150

Dessert

Jimmy Schmidt · Baked Pear with Wildflower Honey, Wine, and Vanilla 151
Larry Forgione · Old-Fashioned Apple and Cranberry Duff 152
Alice Waters · Baked Figs in Red Wine 153

WINTER RECIPES 155

Breakfast

Alice Waters · Banana Pancakes 157
Jimmy Schmidt · Pear, Parsnip, and Potato Pancakes 158
Larry Forgione · Sweet Corn Porridge with Dried Fruits 159

Lunch and Salads

Jimmy Schmidt · Roasted Beets, Endive, and Frisée Salad 160
Jimmy Schmidt · Calamari, White Bean, and Red Lentil Ragout 161
Jimmy Schmidt · Vegetable Black Bean Chili 162
Alice Waters · Smoked Fish and Celery Root Salad 164
Alice Waters · Winter Vegetable Salads 165
Alice Waters · Pasta with Mushrooms, Fennel, and Thyme 166
Larry Forgione · Winter Pear, Endive, and Frisée Salad 167
Larry Forgione · Warm Chicken Salad with Walnut Sherry Vinaigrette 168
Larry Forgione · Seared Sea Scallops with Cranberries and Hickory Nuts 169

Appetizers

Alice Waters · Fish Tartare with Capers, Lemon, and Shallots 170
Larry Forgione · Steamed Mussels with Fennel in an Orange Broth 171
Jimmy Schmidt · Grilled Endive with Parsley and Green Peppercorns 172

Dinner

Larry Forgione · Honey-Glazed Grouper 173
Larry Forgione · Seared Fillets of Pork with Chili Spices and
Maple-Whipped Sweet Potatoes 174
Larry Forgione · Braised Breast of Chicken Smothered with White Beans
and Greens 175
Alice Waters · Bean Soup with Wilted Greens and Rosemary Oil 176
Alice Waters · Braised Duck Legs with Celery Root Purée 178
Alice Waters · Roast Leg of Lamb with Exotic Spices and Yogurt Sauce 180
Jimmy Schmidt · Mahimahi with Grapefruit and Ginger 181
Jimmy Schmidt · Steamed Mussels with Saffron and Spicy Couscous 182
Jimmy Schmidt · Braised Veal Shanks with Celeriac and Mustard 184
Jimmy Schmidt · Swordfish with Coriander and Chives 185

Dessert
Jimmy Schmidt · Cranberry and Orange Soufflé   186
Alice Waters · Pears Poached in Marsala   188
Larry Forgione · Baked Pumpkin and Walnut Pudding   189

BASIC RECIPES   191

TWO-WEEK MENU PLAN   199

APPENDIX   217

INDEX   223

Foreword

———◆———

"If there is a doctor on the plane, would he or she contact one of the flight attendants immediately." I had just settled down as the plane moved along the runway on a flight from New York to Los Angeles. I had opened *Week by Week to a Strong Heart,* a book that we had just finished, and was perusing it for possible quotes for a television interview the following morning. I rose and followed the stewardess to another part of the plane, leaving the book on my seat. Fortunately, the gentleman who had suffered a cardiac arrest responded dramatically to cardiac resuscitation, and within a few minutes was breathing normally, with a regular pulse. It took approximately one and a half hours for him to be removed from the plane (happily in good shape). When I returned to my seat I found my seatmate excitedly holding up my book and announcing that I must write another one. Believing that I had said most of the things that I wanted to say in this as well as in previous books, I told him I didn't think so. But after listening for several minutes to his outline of a book to be written by myself and several of America's best-known chefs, the idea began to take hold. Wouldn't it be nice to explore and clarify some of the myths and misconceptions about diet, antioxidants, garlic, food additives, heart disease, cholesterol, etc., and at the same time demonstrate how people could remain on a low-fat, low-cholesterol diet and still enjoy recipes put together by America's leading chefs?

I still didn't know my seatmate's name. After he had flipped through his Rolodex, called a dozen or more critics, and announced, yes, the chefs would all be willing to participate, I found out that Shep Gordon of Alive Culinary Resources in Los Angeles was the manager of many of the leading chefs in the country. In addition, he was a movie producer and a manager of rock stars. This had indeed been a momentous journey with a fortuitous seat assignment. By the time we reached Los Angeles, Shep had obtained tentative agreements from Alice Waters, Jimmy Schmidt, and Larry Forgione to participate. *Heart-Healthy Cooking for All Seasons* had been born. I look forward to my next "book tour" airplane trip for *Heart-Healthy Cooking for All Seasons.* Anything could happen!

Marvin Moser, M.D.

Introduction

*H*eart-Healthy Cooking for All Seasons is unique. For the first time, an explanation of the scientific facts about heart attack risk factors is presented in a sensible and straightforward manner, coupled with an easy-to-follow program to reduce these factors—a program that includes recipes from three of America's best-known chefs: Alice Waters of Chez Panisse, in Berkeley, California; Larry Forgione of An American Place, in New York City; and Jimmy Schmidt of The Rattlesnake Club, in Detroit, Michigan.

Alice has received numerous awards including the James Beard Special Achievement Award in 1985, and the Best Chef in America and Best Restaurant in America Award from the James Beard Foundation in 1992. She is the author of the *Chez Panisse Menu Cookbook* (Random House, 1982), as well as several other cookbooks. Well-known for her strong position on the seasonal use of fruits and vegetables and a supporter of using antibiotic-free meat and poultry, she is considered among the vanguard of American chefs who care deeply about the environment. As you will see, her beliefs are reflected in her recipes.

Larry also strives to serve only fresh food in his restaurant, with an emphasis on seasonal produce. He, too, has received many honors including the Chef of the Year Award from both the Culinary Institute of America in 1989 and the James Beard Foundation in 1993. *Playboy* magazine selected An American Place as one of America's best restaurants, and the television program *Lifestyles of the Rich and Famous* selected it as one of the world's best.

Jimmy is the author of *Cooking for All Seasons* (Macmillan, 1991) and, like Alice and Larry, has often been honored by his peers—the James Beard Award for Best Chef in the Midwest in 1993 and the Food and Wine Honor Roll of American Chefs are but two of his accolades. As you sample his recipes, you will see why a major magazine listed him as one of the top ten in innovation and trend setting among the nation's chefs.

In *Heart-Healthy Cooking for All Seasons,* facts and myths about heart disease are put in perspective based on up-to-date medical information and my more than forty years of experience as a practicing cardiologist, researcher, and teacher. I have always believed and taught that far more is to be gained by prevention than by the excessive testing and overuse of procedures that are now common practice in cardiology. As the senior medical consultant to the National High Blood Pressure Education Program of the National Heart, Lung and Blood Institute, and as a clinical professor of medicine at the Yale University School of Medicine, I have had the opportunity to be involved in some of the major programs designed to prevent heart disease in the United States. Over the years, it has become increasingly clear that extreme, rigid, or complicated programs do not work for most people and more importantly *are not necessary* to reduce the risk of heart attack or stroke—which explains in large part my involvement in *Heart-Healthy Cooking for All Seasons.* The book presents a program that stresses moderation while making suggestions for what you should do—but also emphasizes what you do *not* have to do to keep heart attack risk factors under control.

This is not a diet book. The word "diet" suggests deprivation. Nor is this a traditional cookbook, although it contains more than a hundred delicious new recipes from Alice, Larry, and Jimmy. It's a book about healthy eating and living without deprivation. We've gotten together to present the real facts about the risks for heart disease and to show you how you can reduce them. By putting into practice the simple concept of "fat budgeting," you will be able to control your fat intake, reduce your weight, and control your cholesterol levels without converting your kitchen into a diet center, turning your pocketbook inside out, or becoming a "cholesterol neurotic."

What About Fat Budgeting?

Almost everyone has to budget their resources: so much for rent, so much for food, so much for education, and so on. If, for example, you spend a lot on entertainment one month, you may have to cut back the next month. This same logic holds true with regulating (or budgeting) your intake of various foods. In this book, we attempt to show you how to do just that: specifically, to budget your fat, cholesterol, and calorie intake so that you can truly enjoy food while adhering to what is considered a balanced, tasty, and nutritious diet. The recipes here include many foods that nowadays are shunned as being "unhealthy"—but if you monitor your intake, they are no less healthful than many other foods.

On these pages, we will demystify the heart attack risk factors and explain how to eat nutritious, great-tasting foods and still maintain a low-fat, low-cholesterol diet essential to any risk-reduction program.

Changing Our Diets

There is little doubt that most of us would be better off eating less fat and fewer foods high in cholesterol. Abundant data exist to prove this point. At the same time, there are scores of programs designed to achieve these goals that advocate rigid diets calling for hard-to-find, difficult-to-prepare foods, and others that recommend unyielding vegetarian regimens. Both approaches too often result in people saying, "The heck with it! I'm not going to do anything."

As a nation, Americans are not quite ready to alter their eating habits drastically. But scientific evidence indicates that *some* changes should be made. We suffer from too many diet-related illnesses not to take action. However, extreme stands generally do not have much lasting success. And, more importantly, they are most often not necessary!

One thing about which I am quite certain is that you do not have to devote a good part of your daily thoughts and activities to rigid dieting, expensive or time-consuming exercise programs and long hours of soul searching in order to reduce your risk of heart disease. I have been amazed at how the media have repeatedly, and often uncritically, embraced and publicized each new "life saving program." These programs often advocate activities that few people have the time, resources or discipline to follow—and most often fail to produce any better results than can be achieved by less restrictive routines.

The latest in the series of miracles is the California lifestyle plan—The Ornish Program. This advocates a vegetarian diet (less than 10 percent of calories as fat and about 5–10 mg of cholesterol per day). This is coupled with an expensive exercise and relaxation program that requires a commitment of 15–20 hours per week.

Yes, a few people can follow this program and benefit is noted in people who already have heart disease, but even the doctors involved admit that it may not be practical. Very few physicians are convinced that all components of the regimen are necessary. Similar results have actually been achieved in other programs that are more practical and can be adhered to by most people.

A good example is a study at St. Thomas' Hospital in London (reported in the medical journal *The Lancet* in March 1992). People with heart disease were placed on a daily diet in which 27 percent of calories came from fat and a total of 100–200 mg of cholesterol were consumed. After three years of this well-tolerated diet 38 percent of the people in the treatment group showed an improvement in coronary artery lesions (compared to only 4 percent in a usual diet group). Progression or worsening of plaques in the arteries occurred in only 15 percent of diet subjects (compared to 46 percent in the non-treated people). Similar results have also been obtained in a Heidelberg, Germany, trial in which dietary fat composed about 20 percent of calories and cholesterol intake was about 200 mg per day.

We recognize the results of these scientific studies in *Heart-Healthy Cooking for All Seasons*. We suggest an intake of 25 percent of calories from fat and about 250 mg of cholesterol—and if a dietary program isn't successful in significantly reducing cholesterol levels, there are now effective and safe medications that can be used along with the diet to lower cholesterol and slow down or prevent progression of artery disease. The use of medication and a practical diet has resulted in a marked reduction in heart attack rates in people at high risk of heart disease.

We will show you why miracle diets and rigid programs don't work. It stands to reason that if the very first "miracle" diet or program had proven effective, there would have been no need for the "new" one that, for the past twenty years or more, has been appearing on the culinary horizon every six to twelve months. It's time to admit that there are no miracles.

We intend to demonstrate how, within the context of the fat-budget concept, you can stay healthy and still eat quite normally by making sensible changes in your diet. Yes, you can include foods such as red meat, cheese, and eggs and still keep your total fat intake below the 25 to 30 percent of total calories advocated by national health care committees. Saturated fat can be kept to about 7 to 8 percent of total calories and cholesterol below 250 mg per day. We call this intelligent eating. "Intelligent" because by following our advice and recipes you can reduce your risk of heart disease and still eat foods that taste good.

The Recipes
Most of the recipes in this book conform to national guidelines for recommended fat and cholesterol intake. For the few that do not, we explain how to budget your fat intake on the days you choose one of these particular recipes or on the day or two after you splurge. After all, when the recipes come from chefs with the stature of Larry Forgione, Jimmy Schmidt, and Alice Waters, they are hard to resist. While most are relatively low in fat and calories, and high in complex carbohydrates and fiber, a few exceed the strict boundaries only because it was necessary to include some extra fat for better taste. Take a look at Larry Forgione's Roast Chicken with Apple-Sage Dressing on page 145 for an example of an over-the-limit recipe. Even without the skin, the per-portion calorie count is 858 and the per-portion fat-gram count is 44! With sensible budgeting on the few days after you eat this meal, you can easily include it, without worry. Remember, we are interested in fine flavor and true enjoyment and we certainly are also aware that a low-fat diet is a healthy diet. We will detail a program that includes your usual foods and a daily pick of the chefs' recipes— and keeps the lid on cholesterol and fat.

We will also address the confusing area of how diet may or may not control blood pressure and elevated cholesterol levels. Our answers may be surprising, as both these issues have been distorted by countless articles and books that have done more to confuse the public than enlighten it.

Our book can become a quick and easy reference guide for the home cook. The information contained here is pertinent to nearly everyone, whether you are concerned with learning more about the primary risk factors for heart disease and high blood pressure or the dangers of smoking, obesity, and diabetes, or just how to control your blood cholesterol levels. Equally important (and let's face it, a lot more fun!) are the recipes. Because we all believe that a healthful diet need not be dreary or gimmicky, the chefs have agreed to join forces with me to share their creativity and extensive culinary knowledge. You will be surprised to learn that you can eat your cake, have a steak or veal shank, and still not violate the rules of "heart healthy" eating. For example, look at Alice Waters' recipe for Grilled Steak with Gremolata on page 138. There certainly is not so much fat or cholesterol in this to suggest that you avoid it. Or look at Jimmy Schmidt's recipe on page 184 for Braised Veal Shanks with Celeriac and Mustard. You can eat these foods without guilt.

We hope this book will become a trusted friend in the kitchen that you will turn to and use time and again. The recipes are organized seasonally so that you can take full advantage of the foods that are freshest and best at any given time of year. We believe that by eating fresh food grown in its natural season, you are contributing to your good health and well-being, and getting the most out of what you eat. Good health, full enjoyment, and the reduction of anxiety about what we eat is what we hope to bring to you.

ABOUT WEIGHT

———◦◦◦———

With more than 30 million Americans considered overweight and in need of some program to help them lose weight, it's important to understand why we gain weight and why being heavy is a major risk factor for heart disease and other illnesses. Perhaps it's even more important to understand that losing weight and maintaining a reasonable norm is not as hard as many people have been led to believe—and doesn't require rigid dieting or depriving yourself of delicious foods. It does mean that you'll probably have to exercise more and make some adjustments in your calorie intake, especially as this relates to fatty foods.

Integrating a lower-fat and lower-calorie diet into your daily life does not mean a life sentence of dreary dieting. On the contrary, you can enjoy lots of appetizing low-fat, low-calorie dishes as well as some that are not in this category—if you budget your intake.

FAT BUDGETING

What exactly does "fat budgeting" mean? Most experts agree that we would be healthier if we kept our total daily fat intake at about 25 percent or less of total calories instead of the current level of about 35 percent. *(For example—on a 2,000-calorie intake, only about 500 calories or less should come from fat.* Since 1 g of fat = 9 calories, total fat intake should be limited to less than 55 g. Many people are aware of this recommendation; the average amount of fat in the typical American diet has actually decreased from 42 percent in 1960—but we have a way to go. To achieve the desired goal does not mean, however, that you have to watch your fat intake with each and every meal. If you go over the limit on Monday and Tuesday, be more careful on Wednesday, Thursday, and Friday.

Most of the recipes in this book are designed to help you keep your fat intake (especially saturated fat) within acceptable limits. They are different from the creamy, rich, buttery foods of yesteryear—and in many instances, better tasting. Some recipes may contain more than the suggested quota of fat and this is where the fat budgeting system is put to work.

As we go along with each set of recipes, we'll show you how to do this, and in the Two-Week Menu Plan (page 199) we'll be specific about achieving a proper balance of fat intake and enjoyable eating. After a while, budgeting will become second nature, and in a short time you will lose some of your craving for those foods that you once thought were essential for eating enjoyment. Some dishes are deceptively high in fat. For example, look at Jimmy Schmidt's recipe for Sliced Tomatoes, Grilled Onion, and Fried Basil Salad on page 86. This simple-sounding recipe, so good when tomatoes and basil are in season in high summer, is quite high in fat because of the relatively large amount of olive oil it uses. But of the 20.7g (grams) of fat (186 fat calories) per serving, only 2.8 are saturated, and so the salad probably poses no increased risk of a heart attack. (Saturated fat is the major contributor to increased cholesterol levels.) Nevertheless, fat intake should be monitored (or budgeted) in relation to the rest of the food you eat that day. Another example of a recipe that is high in fat is Alice Waters' Smoked Fish and Celery Root Salad on page 164, with 21 g of fat per serving (189 fat calories). Again, the olive oil accounts for the fat content—but a high olive oil intake does not increase heart attack risk (see Saturated Fats and Trans-Fatty Acids). Enjoy this for lunch but watch your total fat and calorie intake that evening and you will be well within your "budget"—even if you're trying to lose weight.

SATURATED FATS AND TRANS-FATTY ACIDS

• Some fat intake is necessary for the body to manufacture hormones and cell membranes.

• Fats in foods are necessary to carry vitamins A, E, and K in the bloodstream. Fats are transported in the blood with proteins, so-called lipo (fat) proteins. For example, *high-* and *low-density lipoproteins* (HDLs and LDLs) describe types of fat that are combined with proteins in the blood (see Cholesterol: The Myths and the Facts, beginning on page 25).

    A. Saturated fats

        1. Are solid at room temperature.

        2. Almost always come from animal sources (butter, cheese, milk, meats, or poultry with skin). Exceptions are palm and coconut oils and hydrogenated oils such as solid vegetable shortening.

        3. Interfere with the enzyme systems that help to remove cholesterol from the blood. As cholesterol levels rise, heart attack risk increases.

        4. Have a greater effect on raising blood cholesterol levels than dietary cholesterol itself.

    B. Monosaturated fats

        1. Are liquid at room temperature.

        2. Are found in olive and peanut oils.

        3. Are high in calories but may actually reduce blood cholesterol levels when used to replace saturated fats and do not increase the risk for heart disease. (People who live in countries with low heart attack rates, such as Italy and France, use lots of olive oil, which may in part account for this phenomenon.)

    C. Polyunsaturated fats

        1. Are liquid even at cold temperatures.

        2. Are found in soybeans and soybean, corn, safflower, and sesame oils, as well as in fish oil.

        3. Some may reduce heart attack risk by reducing the tendency of blood to clot.

• Hydrogenation is a process used to make liquid fats more solid and more stable.

    The most common example of hydrogenation is the conversion of soft margarine to a semisolid state. The process increases the percentage of saturated fat and trans-fatty acids, which may increase the risk of heart disease. If you use margarine, corn oil margarine in tub form is best. The fat that results when this type of oil is partially hydrogenated does not raise cholesterol levels or increase heart attack risk. *Soft* corn oil margarine is even better. Some recent studies suggest that a high intake of hydrogenated or "stick" margarines may be just as bad for you as eating lots of butter—on balance, however, margarine is probably to be preferred. Most of us do not use enough of these kinds of margarine to increase our intake of trans-fatty acids to an important extent.

What Is Obesity?

About 40 to 50 percent of Americans are more than 20–25 percent heavier than their ideal weight and are considered overweight. Ten percent are more than 30 percent above ideal weight and are considered obese. Ideal weight is determined from long-term epidemiologic studies showing that people who exceed certain weights are more susceptible to many diseases, such as high blood pressure, diabetes, heart attacks, and certain types of cancer. In addition, several forms of arthritis (for example, gout and osteoarthritis) are more common in people who are heavy. In other words, there is a major incentive to keep as close to ideal weight as possible. But what is ideal weight? Most of us can determine if we are overweight simply by looking in a mirror, but if in doubt, there are several simple ways to calculate ideal weight. For instance, look at A Simple Method to Figure Your Ideal Weight to determine *approximately* what you should ideally weigh. These weights vary a little depending on body type and age, but they are good guidelines. Another more accurate way to determine whether you are too heavy is to use what is called the *body mass index*. This may appear to be complicated but Chart 2 is really quite easy to use.

A SIMPLE METHOD TO FIGURE YOUR IDEAL WEIGHT

Anyone who weighs about 20 to 30 percent more than his or her "ideal weight" is considered overweight. As noted below, a woman who is 5 feet 5 inches tall should weigh *about* 125 pounds. If she weighs 25 to 30 pounds more than this, or approximately 150 to 155 pounds, she is considered overweight. There are more complicated and probably more accurate methods of calculating desirable weights by using what is called the *body mass index* (see Body Weight in Pounds According to Height and BMI), but the following will give you a good idea of what you should weigh *ideally*.

WOMEN: Allow 100 pounds for the first 5 feet of height: 100
              Add 5 pounds for each additional inch of height (25 pounds for a 5'5" woman):   +25
              Ideal body weight for a 5'5" woman: 125

MEN: Allow 106 pounds for the first 5 feet of height: 106
              Add 6 pounds for each additional inch of height (72 pounds for a 6' man):   +72
              Ideal body weight for a 6' man: 178

Being overweight or obese is detrimental to psychological health. The process of trying to control weight becomes a vicious cycle. Some obesity results from psychological problems—people overeat for gratification or out of boredom or fear; once they become overweight, their self-esteem may decrease, making it even harder to lose weight or, if they lose it, to maintain an ideal weight. Some obesity is hereditary. An obesity gene has been discovered. Mutations, or changes, in this gene may alter the way in which parts of the brain respond to hunger sensations and may explain why some people can eat and eat and never feel full. It is extremely difficult for them to limit their calorie intake. Those who have a family trait must be particularly careful about limiting total calorie intake in themselves and their children. A fat adolescent usually becomes a fat adult, so paying attention to this is particularly important.

Once the number of fat cells in the body increases, as they do in overweight teenagers, it becomes more difficult to lose weight. Occasionally weight gain or inability to lose weight results from an underactive thyroid gland—food is metabolized at a slower rate and weight increases without an increase in calorie intake—but this is an uncommon cause of being overweight.

BODY WEIGHT IN POUNDS ACCORDING TO HEIGHT AND BMI

This measurement is accurate because it considers whether someone has a small or large body frame. People with a body mass index (BMI) of more than 30 are considered obese. They are overweight if the BMI is between 27 and 30, and of desirable weight if the BMI is between 23 and 27. For example, according to the table below, a 5 foot 5 inch (65-inch) tall woman (1) who weighs 162 pounds has a body mass index (BMI) of 27. She would be considered overweight but not obese. A 6 foot 1 inch (73-inch) tall man (2) who weighs 228 pounds has a body mass index (BMI) of more than 30 and would be considered obese.

It may seem unimportant to get involved in definitions of ideal weight, overweight, or obesity, but knowing where you stand is helpful in setting targets for weight loss or keeping an ideal weight. (You just have to check it once.)

	BODY MASS INDEX (KG/M^*)												
	19	20	21	22	23	24	25	26	27	28	29	30	35	40
HEIGHT (IN.) BODY WEIGHT (LB)														
58	91	96	100	105	110	115	119	124	129	134	138	143	167	191
59	94	99	104	109	114	119	124	128	133	138	143	148	173	198
60	97	102	107	112	118	123	128	133	138	143	148	153	179	204
61	100	106	111	116	122	127	132	137	143	148	153	158	185	211
62	104	109	115	120	126	131	136	142	147	153	158	164	191	218
63	107	113	118	124	130	135	141	146	152	158	163	169	197	225
64	110	116	122	128	134	140	145	151	157	163	169	174	204	232
65	114	120	126	132	138	144	150	156	162	168	174	180	210	240
66	118	124	130	136	142	148	155	161	167	173	179	186	216	247
67	121	127	134	140	146	153	159	166	172	178	185	191	223	255
68	125	131	138	144	151	158	164	171	177	184	190	197	230	262
69	128	135	142	149	155	162	169	176	182	189	196	203	236	270
70	132	139	146	153	160	167	174	181	188	195	202	207	243	278
71	136	143	150	157	165	172	179	186	193	200	208	215	250	286
72	140	147	154	162	169	177	184	191	199	206	213	221	258	294
73	144	151	159	166	174	182	189	197	204	212	219	227	265	302
74	148	155	163	171	179	186	194	202	210	218	225	233	272	311
75	152	160	168	176	184	192	200	208	216	224	232	240	279	319
76	156	164	172	180	189	197	205	213	221	230	238	246	287	328

*Measured as kilograms (2.2 lb.) per meter square (m^2).

Obesity takes several forms. The type of fat distribution may affect the risk for heart disease. Men begin to develop a pot belly or abdominal obesity ("apple-shaped" obesity) as they age, usually around thirty-five or forty. This type of obesity increases heart attack risk. There are also some women who develop abdominal or trunkal obesity and, like men with abdominal obesity, will have elevated cholesterol levels and will be more susceptible to diabetes than women who simply gain weight in the thighs and buttocks. The latter "pear-shaped" obesity is the more common type in women (a relatively thin upper torso and heavy buttocks and thighs). If the ratio of the waist to hip circumference is more than 1.0 in a man or 0.8 in a woman, it is an indication of an increased risk for vascular disease and diabetes. (For example, a 42-inch waist and 40-inch hip measurement in a male gives a ratio of more than 1.0 and is not ideal.) Abdominal fat is more easily mobilized than fat in other places. It is absorbed into the liver where it may not be effectively metabolized and excreted; it enters the bloodstream as increased cholesterol and triglycerides, another fatty substance (see Cholesterol: The Myths and the Facts). In addition, insulin metabolism is adversely affected in people with excessive amounts of abdominal fat, hence the increased chance of developing diabetes.

Even if you were a thin young adult, it is important to watch your weight when you get to be "thirtysomething." Calorie needs decrease about 2 percent every decade after age thirty or forty, and it's easy to let pounds creep onto your body, especially since many people decrease their physical activity at these ages. This explains why so many people in their fifties and sixties complain that they "don't eat a thing" and still gain or can't lose weight.

Why Some People Gain Weight and Others Do Not
Some of us are lucky. We can eat more than 3,000 calories a day and not gain a pound. Others *look* at a calorie and add a pound. Often the reason for this is that the heavy person produced more fat cells than were necessary during childhood. Fat is easily stored in these cells. Whether this is genetic or due to "overfeeding" as a child is not firmly established, but as we have noted, overweight adolescents tend to become overweight adults. It is a good idea to instill good nutritional habits in children and teens even if there is no family history of obesity or diabetes. Doing so will help young and middle-aged adults control their weight more easily. This is important, since obesity presents more risk for this age group than it does for the elderly.

How to Lose Weight
Losing weight is a matter of arithmetic. If you consume more calories than you expend, or use up, you gain weight. If you burn up more than you take in, you lose weight. One pound of weight is lost for every 3,500 calories expended over and above what is taken in. For example, if you normally consume 2,500 calories a day and reduce that amount to 2,000 a day for one week, you will lose one pound (500 calories/day × 7 = 3,500 calories = 1 pound). If you reduce your intake by 300 calories a day and burn up an extra 200 calories a day by doing some additional exercise, you'll accomplish the same thing. You may even do better than the arithmetic suggests—exercise not only consumes calories, it helps to speed up the rate that the body burns calories, even at rest. So you get a double bonus.

The box How Many Calories? tells you how to figure out just how many calories you need to maintain your weight. Table 1 illustrates just how many calories are used by various exercises. Note that you do not have to be a "fitness nut" to use up calories—but also note that losing weight by exercise alone can be difficult. Just eating a hamburger on a bun and drinking a Coke, for example, adds up to about 600 calories. You would have to play tennis

HOW MANY CALORIES?

The key questions are: How many calories do I need or require to keep my weight stable so that I won't gain? and, If I've lost weight, how can I keep from gaining it back? There is a simple formula to help answer these questions. This applies to men and women approximately between ages thirty and fifty-five. Calorie needs are about 10 to 20 percent less for older individuals.

Take your *ideal* weight: for example, a 5-foot 10-inch man weighing 166 pounds.

If *sedentary,* multiply 166 (his weight) by *13*: he would need *about* 2,158 calories a day to maintain this weight

If *moderately active,* multiply 166 by *15*: he would need *about* 2,490 calories a day to maintain this weight

If *very active,* multiply 166 by *17*: he would need 2,822 calories a day to maintain this weight

If this man were to take in more than the calculated number of calories, he would gain weight; if less, he would probably lose weight. Remember, a sedentary person whose calorie requirements are 2,150 calories might be able to take in as many as 2,300 to 2,400 calories if he or she becomes more active and uses up the extra calories by exercising.

for one and a half hours or walk at a vigorous pace of 3 miles per hour (mph) for two hours to burn these calories. Weight loss usually requires a combination of less food and more exercise. See Sample Calorie Targets for Losing Weight (page 16) for examples of calorie targets that result in weight loss.

This all sounds easy—just use up more than you take in—and it is for some people. Yet, millions of Americans battle with their weight daily, weekly, yearly. Thirty years ago, a physician who was an expert in treating obesity summarized his results in treating people who were more than 40 to 50 pounds overweight. "Most obese persons will not stay in treatment for obesity," he said. "Of those who stay in treatment, most will not lose weight, and of those who do lose weight, most will regain it."

This gloomy statement was uttered in 1958 and there are still many who believe it today. But it doesn't have to be so, not if you are patient and use common sense.

"Quick Fix" or Gimmicky Rigid Diets Don't Work

Losing a pound or two a week sounds like a slow, tortuous way to lose weight and frankly, most Americans ignore the logic of it. We are impatient people who subscribe to miracle diets as soon as the newest one appears on the horizon in the form of a new book or article in a women's magazine, or as promoted by a fast-talking "expert" on television talk shows. We want instant results, with someone telling us exactly what to do. The truth is that most miracle diets don't work because they don't change behavior and long-term eating patterns. Follow-up studies demonstrate that most people who lose weight by following either very low calorie diets, liquid diets, or diets that require a major change in the types of food "allowed" usually gain back the weight in a short period of time. For instance, patients who

TABLE 1

CALORIES USED BY EXERCISING*

ACTIVITY	APPROXIMATE CALORIES BURNED PER HALF-HOUR
NORMAL ACTIVITIES	
CLEANING WINDOWS	130
GARDENING	110
MOPPING FLOORS	130
MOWING LAWN (POWER MOWER)	125
SITTING/CONVERSING	40
VACUUMING	130
MODERATE EXERCISE	
BICYCLING (6 MPH)	135
BOWLING	135
PLAYING GOLF (USING POWER CART)	100
PLAYING GOLF (PULLING CART)	135
PLAYING VOLLEYBALL	175
ROLLER SKATING	175
SQUARE DANCING	175
SWIMMING (¼ MPH)	150
WALKING (1 MPH)	65
WALKING (3 MPH)	140
VIGOROUS EXERCISE	
BICYCLING (11 MPH)	225
HILL CLIMBING (100 FT/HR)	245
ICE SKATING (10 MPH)	200
JOGGING (5 MPH)	265
PLAYING SQUASH OR HANDBALL	300
PLAYING TENNIS	210
RUNNING (8 MPH)	360
SKIING (20 MPH)	300
WALKING (4 MPH)	195

This will give you some idea of how many calories are used up by various activities. As you look at the recipes in this book and review your total daily calorie intake, you should get a good idea of just how much exercise is necessary to balance out any excess calories.

consume a low-calorie liquid formula diet, even under medical supervision, may lose approximately 30 to 40 pounds during a three- to four-month period. But they regain about 50 to 65 percent or more of this loss during the following year. Yo-yo dieting has been shown over and over again to be ineffective and what's more, it may backfire. The dieter may end up weighing *more* than he or she did before beginning the first diet. When you go on a very low calorie diet (for example, less than about 1,000 calories/day), your body's metabolic rate decreases (you burn up calories more slowly as a protective mechanism). When you resume a more normal caloric intake, your body continues to use up calories at a lower rate for a while and you gain weight. One important point: In any weight-loss program, the first 3 to 4 pounds lost are most likely fluid and reappear when you go back to "regular" eating. Don't be misled into believing that you've lost fat.

Some people who are seriously or morbidly overweight (more than 80 to 100 percent over ideal weight) and have diabetes or severe hypertension may have to get started on weight loss under medical supervision. In some cases, this may mean going on a liquid formula diet (about 800 or fewer calories per day). Clearly more weight will come off following one of these diets than it will following a 1,200- to 1,500-calorie-a-day intake, but there is also the danger of developing gallstones and of harmful "binge" eating even while on the controlled regimen. This approach might, however, be useful for a month or two. It is easier and wiser over the long term to follow the program outlined on the following pages.

SAMPLE CALORIE TARGETS FOR LOSING WEIGHT

A. A 5-foot 5-inch, 140-pound sedentary woman who wishes to lose 15 pounds to achieve her ideal weight of 125 pounds:

    1. Begins to walk for one hour a day at about 2 miles per hour.

    Extra calories consumed: about $110/day \times 7 = 770/week$.

    2. Reduces her calorie intake from 2,500/day to 1,700/day (a relatively easy target).

    Change in calorie intake:

    800 fewer calories/day

    5,600 fewer calories/week

    Total calorie difference (including exercise results): 6,370, or a loss of almost 2 pounds/week.

    Calculation: 3,500 calories = 1 pound

                      6,370 calories = 1.82 pounds

B. A 6-foot, 195-pound moderately active man who wishes to lose about 15 pounds to achieve his ideal weight of 180:

    1. Uses a stationary bicycle for thirty minutes a day in addition to his usual twice-weekly game of tennis.

    Extra calories consumed: $100\ cal/day \times 7 = 700\ calories/week$.

    2. Reduces his calorie intake from 3,000/day to 2,200/day by reducing portions of food by half (without a rigid diet).

    Change in calorie intake:

    800 fewer calories/day

    5,600 fewer calories/week

    Total calorie difference (including exercise results): 6,300, or a loss of almost 2 pounds/week

    Calculation: 3,500 calories = 1 pound

                      6,300 calories = 1.8 pounds

It Takes Common Sense

The commonsense approach to eating for long-term weight loss, weight control, and reduction of your risk for heart and other diseases is: 1) to reduce the overall number of calories you consume over time, and 2) to monitor your intake of fat so that no more than 25 percent of your calories come from fat—and no more than 7 to 8 percent come from saturated fat. See the box How To Figure Fat Intake, for information. Remember, each gram of fat supplies more than twice the number of calories as a gram of protein or carbohydrate (9 calories in a gram of fat compared to 4 in a gram of protein or carbohydrates).

How to Figure Fat Intake

1. *Total fat-calorie intake* should be limited to 500 calories (25 percent of total) on a 2,000-calorie/day intake. Since each gram of fat generates 9 calories, this translates to about 55 g of fat/day.*

2. *Saturated fat* should be limited to about 7 to 8 percent of total calories. On a 2,000-calorie/day intake, about 140 to 160 calories should come from saturated fat—or less than 20 g of saturated fat.

3. *Adjust these numbers for total calories.* For example, on a weight loss program of 1,200 calories/day, 300 calories, or 27 g of total fat with less than 100 calories or about 10–11 g of saturated fat, would be ideal.

Remember, these numbers are not etched in granite; they should be used as guidelines, not as rigid targets.

Daily calorie needs = 2000 calories
  25% of 2000 = 500
  500/9 = 55 g

Table 2 gives you more details about recommended fat and saturated fat intake levels with various calorie intakes. It may appear complicated to have to figure all of this out, but most of us can get a general idea of the approximate amount of fat in various foods within a short time—it never has to be an exact count. After the initial period of "awareness," it is not difficult to do the proper budgeting.

You may be surprised to know that many of the "forbidden meats" (which do contain saturated fat) can become part of any low-fat diet. As you will see when we analyze the recipes from Alice, Jimmy, and Larry, there are quite a few meat dishes. Budget them into your daily menus and enjoy. Just to show you that they are not as harmful as you have been led to believe, let's look at the calorie, fat, and saturated fat contents of some meats and poultry (Tables 3 and 4).

While a high *percentage* of fat is derived from calories in the meats listed in Table 3, you can see in a minute that even on a 1,500-calorie intake with a maximum prudent intake of about 375 calories from total fat and about 120 calories from saturated fat, you can have a 4- to 6-ounce steak without concern. And if you have a larger one once in a while, it also doesn't jeopardize your program. But the word "budget" comes up again—you may have to limit the fat calories from other foods for the next day or so if you go overboard with an

TABLE 2

HOW TO FIGURE YOUR FAT BUDGET BY CALORIE LEVELS

APPROXIMATE ESTIMATED TOTAL DAILY CALORIE INTAKE*	TOTAL FAT CALORIES (IDEALLY, 25% AS TOTAL FAT)†	GRAMS OF FAT	SATURATED FAT CALORIES (IDEALLY, 7% TO 8% AS SATURATED FAT)
1,000	250	28	72
1,200	300	33	90
1,500	375	43	108
1,800	450	50	135
2,000	500	55	145
2,500	625	69	180
2,800	700	78	198
3,000	750	83	216

NOTE: *Most food labels list the total amount of fat in grams and the amount of calories as fat. The number of grams × 9 = the number of calories.*

If your daily calorie requirements, based on ideal weight, are 1,800 (or 1,800 × 7 = 12,600/week), and you binge over a weekend, using up 6,000 calories over the two days, watch your intake the other five days. The same principles apply to fat. If, on the same total calorie intake (12,600/week with 3,150 as fat), you have a piece of pie with ice cream, two hot dogs, and some other high-fat foods on one or two days, using up 1,500 fat calories of your weekly total of 3,150, just be careful for the rest of the week. Budgeting does work and is easy if you set your mind to following the concept.

†*Also remember that if you exceed these guidelines once in a while, you can make up for it later by budgeting your food intake, primarily your intake of fat.*

8-ounce special. Let's look again at recipes on pages 138 and 184 which include beef and veal. With the first, Grilled Steak with Gremolata from Alice Waters, the total fat of 12.9 g per serving may appear to be high and the total fat calories of about 115 are more than one third of the total of 281 calories per serving (with 4.8 g, or 43.2 calories, of saturated fat), but these can certainly fit into your fat budget. When we review Jimmy Schmidt's Braised Veal Shank with Celeriac and Mustard, we see that the total calories per serving come in at 433—and the total fat is 17.1 g per serving, or about 153 calories, with saturated fat just over 3 g, or 27 calories, per serving. This level of intake is within a desired range—even if you are on a limited intake of only 1,800 calories a day.

It is of interest now to take a look at Table 4. We're told to eat lots of fish and poultry on a low-fat, low-cholesterol diet—and that's good advice—which is why many of the recipes in this book contain these ingredients. Fish is a good source of protein, vitamins, and, importantly, unsaturated fat; chicken is also low in saturated fat—*if you do not eat the skin.* But as you can see, many chicken dishes (fried or with skin) actually contain more fat and saturated fat than beef. Factor this into your food choices.

To reiterate: Whether you're trying to lose weight or just trying to maintain your present weight and stay healthy, a balanced diet should contain:

1. Less than 25 percent of calories as total fat.

2. About 7 to 8 percent of calories as saturated fat.

TABLE 3

CALORIES, TOTAL FAT, AND SATURATED FAT IN MEAT

Although even lean cuts of beef or pork may derive a relatively high percentage of their calories from fat, the *total amount* in small portions (4 to 6 ounces) is not great enough to warrant their prohibition from a low-fat diet.

	APPROXIMATE TOTAL IN CALORIES	GRAMS TOTAL FAT	CALORIES FROM TOTAL FAT	GRAMS SATURATED FAT	CALORIES FROM SATURATED FAT
LEAN CUTS					
SIRLOIN STEAK	230–350	10–14	90–126	4–6	36–54
TOP ROUND	220–330	7–10	63–90	3–4	27–36
TENDERLOIN PORK	220–345	11–16	99–144	4–6	36–54
CANADIAN BACON	200–310	9–14	81–126	3–4	27–36
TENDERLOIN	180–280	5–8	45–72	1–2	9–18
LEAN CANNED HAM	135–210	5–8	45–72	1–2	9–18

NOTE: *Any of the above foods can easily be fit into a daily total of 500 fat calories a day (or a 2,000-calorie-a-day total). For example, 4 to 6 ounces of lean steak contains not more than about 125 calories as fat calories.*

Eating a steak or some ham will not even upset your saturated fat budget if, for example, about 150 saturated fat calories are allowed in an 1,800- to 2,000-a-day intake. Not more than about 55 calories are derived from saturated fat in the same portion of steak.

Eat these and all red meats sparingly and avoid or eat very sparingly the really fatty meats such as bacon, sausages, hot dogs, etc. (Also be aware that any processed foods may contain too much sodium if you are on a low-sodium diet.)

3. Not more than 250 mg/day* of cholesterol (more about this in Chapter 2).

In addition:

4. Fifteen to 20 percent of the calories should be as protein (fish, poultry, dairy products, skim milk, low-fat cheeses, lean meat, peas and beans); and

5. At least 50 to 55 percent should be as carbohydrates (pasta, rice, cereals, grains, vegetables, bread, beans, fruits, etc.)

If you're trying to lose weight, you will be emphasizing a lower calorie intake, which automatically will mean fewer calories as fat.

As we review the recipes in this book, we will explain the components of various foods and how to accomplish a balanced food intake without having to take a course in nutrition. If you're doing this already, that's fine; just enjoy the new recipes from the chefs. But if you have to change your eating habits, remember that you should change them forever. As

The abbreviation "mg" stands for "milligram." There are 1,000 mg in 1 g.

TABLE 4
APPROXIMATE NUMBER OF CALORIES AND AMOUNTS OF TOTAL FAT AND SATURATED FAT IN POULTRY

	TOTAL CALORIES	GRAMS OF TOTAL FAT	TOTAL CALORIES FROM FAT	GRAMS OF SATURATED FAT	TOTAL CALORIES FROM SATURATED FAT
CHICKEN BREAST (4 OUNCES)					
FRIED WITH SKIN	251	10	90	3	27
ROASTED WITHOUT SKIN	186	4	36	1	9
FAST FOOD, FRIED	279	15	135	4	36
TURKEY (5 OUNCES)					
WHITE MEAT WITHOUT SKIN	182	4	36	2	18
DARK MEAT WITH SKIN	263	14	126	4	36
TURKEY ROLL	169	8	72	2	18
DUCK (4 OUNCES)					
ROASTED WITH SKIN	385	32	288	11	99
WITHOUT SKIN	228	13	117	5	45

we've pointed out, this does not necessarily mean turning your kitchen into "diet central" or staying away from the kinds of good foods that we'll describe later on. Happily, there is no need to go out and buy faddish foods that must be eaten in some magical sequence. Instead, concentrate on fresh vegetables and fruits (especially when they're in season), grains, low-fat meats and dairy products, and herbs and spices. Obviously, cut back on foods high in animal fat and butterfat, and, if your blood pressure is elevated or you have heart disease, those high in sodium. Processed foods, canned soups, pickles, and junk foods are the worst offenders. Furthermore, because you are not going to be eating foods from our recipes alone, we'll discuss later how to combine these with your "usual" breakfast, lunch, or dinner, and keep your fat and calorie intake in check (see pages 199–212).

Following are two examples of how to integrate the chefs' recipes with everyday foods. The Two-Week Meal Plan (pages 199–211) provides other examples.

Getting Started
Commit yourself to the fat-budget concept. This means learning which foods are high in fat and which are not and then cutting back on those that are. But, as we've mentioned several times, don't panic if one day you eat a steak or scoop of Häagen-Dazs ice cream—just be careful about your fat intake for the next few days.

Remember that fat budgeting means stretching out your fat grams (and calories) over about a week's time. We all have "bad" days when all we can manage to eat are high-fat foods available from a coffee cart or airport snack shop. When this happens, adjust your fat-

TABLE 5

DAY I

BREAKFAST	LUNCH	DINNER
6 ounces orange juice; 1 cup corn flakes with 1 cup skim or 1% milk; black coffee	*Tuna fish sandwich; coffee with or without skim or 1% milk or diet soda; 10–15 grapes or 1 apple*	*Tossed salad with oil and vinegar; Alice Waters' Roast Leg of Lamb with Exotic Spices and Yogurt Sauce; roll with 1 teaspoon tub margarine; 1 cup of rice and about ½ cup of green beans; black coffee or tea; 1 apple or pear*
TOTAL CALORIES: 282	400	1,020
TOTAL FAT: 3.0 g	14.8 g	33 g
WITH 1% MILK; *LESS WITH SKIM*		
SATURATED FAT: 1.7 g	2.8 g	8.3 g
CHOLESTEROL: 10 mg	35 mg	156 mg

TOTAL CALORIES PER DAY I: 1,702
TOTAL FAT PER DAY I: 50.8 g
TOTAL SATURATED FAT PER DAY I: 12.8 g
TOTAL CHOLESTEROL PER DAY I: 201 mg
These values are within the limits of the fat-budget plan and allow for a glass of wine at dinner (75 calories), an apple as a snack (60–70 calories), and some sherbet for dessert (130 calories).

DAY II SUNDAY

BREAKFAST	LUNCH	DINNER
Orange juice; Jimmy Schmidt's Pear, Parsnip, and Potato Pancake; black coffee or coffee with skim milk	*Turkey sandwich with 1 teaspoon mayonnaise; black coffee or with skim milk or tea or diet soda; 1 apple*	*Tossed salad with oil and vinegar; 2 cups pasta with red sauce and Parmesan cheese; two gingersnaps or graham crackers; black coffee or with skim milk or tea (with or without sugar)*
TOTAL CALORIES: 600	525	720
TOTAL FAT: 8.5 g	9 g	19 g
SATURATED FAT: 4.1 g	2.4 g	3.5 g
CHOLESTEROL: 63 mg	50 mg	15 mg

TOTAL CALORIES PER DAY II: 1,845
TOTAL FAT PER DAY II: 36.5 g
TOTAL SATURATED FAT PER DAY II: 10 g
TOTAL CHOLESTEROL PER DAY II: 128 mg
As you can see, you are within your budget. But if you do go over the limit with an extra dessert, an ice cream cone, or a high-calorie bedtime snack, just eat less the next day.

gram intake during the rest of the week so that you do not exceed it in any given week. The two-week meal plan that we outline later on shows you exactly how this works.

Deciding to change your eating habits as a means to a healthier life and as a way to control obesity or keep your weight stable is just one step. Acting on the decision is another. I have seen many patients who simply cannot stay on a reasonable program. If you have to lose weight, begin by being completely honest with yourself about the number of calories you consume, your level of activity, and your ability to lose weight. There is a big difference between different people. For example, a mildly obese 5-foot woman who is moderately active might burn up approximately 1,500 calories a day. If she reduces her caloric intake to 1,000 calories, she will lose about a pound a week (500 calories/day × 7 = 3,500 calories = 1 pound). By contrast, a taller, heavier woman who normally burns about 2,500 calories a day will lose far more weight in a week on a 1,000-calorie-a-day diet (or a 1,300-calorie intake plus an extra 300 calories used up by additional exercise). The box below highlights some of the problems that people who are trying to lose weight must face.

QUANTITY CONTROL—IT COUNTS!

Portions and quantity do count if you're trying to lose weight. I always tell patients to reduce the quantity of food by half and still eat the things they enjoy. If cookies are your problem, eat four or five a week instead of ten or fifteen. Eat five or ten slices of bread a week instead of ten to twenty, or one small piece of cake instead of two. Even a candy bar won't hurt once in a while. And remember, 6 to 8 ounces have more calories than 3 to 4 ounces of the *same* food. This is an obvious point, but one that is too often ignored.

Losing weight should not be handled as a one-shot program. Just as we keep a lifelong "eye" on high blood pressure and diabetes, we should watch our weight throughout our lives, since maintaining ideal weight is one of the best ways to slow down the process of atherosclerosis, or hardening of the arteries. This is especially important if someone has been markedly obese and loses weight. Any major loss of weight may actually result in a reversal of some of the changes of "hardening of the arteries." We often wonder why it is some people just can't lose weight, or for that matter, stop smoking until after they have had a heart attack. Don't let that happen to you. Hopefully the recipes in this book and our suggestions about fat budgeting will help you to keep your weight down and to do something to prevent trouble.

Now for Specifics

On pages 199 through 212 we show you how to use our program over a two-week period of time and integrate at least one of the chefs' recipes each day into your usual eating pattern. As you can see, calories can be kept within a target range, and total and saturated fat as well as cholesterol intake can be controlled.

The specific program presented is suitable for a middle-aged woman who is 5 feet 5 inches tall, weighs about 125 pounds, is moderately active, and wishes to maintain her present weight. It is equally appropriate for a man who is 6 feet tall, is sedentary, weighs about 175 pounds, and is not trying to lose weight.

Daily requirements

Total calorie intake: Usually between 1,750 and 2,200 calories/day
Total fat intake: Usually under 500 calories, or 55 g/day
Total saturated fat intake: Usually less than 175 calories/day
Total cholesterol intake: Usually less than 250 to 275 mg/day

(Note: Amounts of food should be adjusted if an overweight man or woman wishes to lose weight. The two-week plan also presents examples of how this can be accomplished.)

Cholesterol:
The Myths and
the Facts

*C*holesterol is the buzz word of the decade. Everyone who reads this book probably knows his or her cholesterol level, and while there is no question that having an elevated blood cholesterol level may increase your risk of developing heart disease, I believe that far too much emphasis has been put on this particular risk factor. In recent years, I have also become concerned that the national guidelines for cholesterol screening and treatment are confusing.

The near obsession with the "cholesterol crusade" continues to cause undue anxiety in too many people, especially younger women who are otherwise healthy and people over the age of seventy-five or eighty who have no evidence of heart disease. Isn't it ridiculous for an eighty-year-old person to worry about eating an egg now and then, or a healthy, thin young woman of forty or forty-five with no risk factors other than a slightly elevated blood cholesterol level to be losing sleep because she ate a bowl of ice cream? We're going to show you how you can put the whole cholesterol story in perspective and when you should really become concerned about it.

Concern over cholesterol *is* appropriate; there is good evidence from many large population studies that people with *lower* levels in their blood have *less* vascular disease. Data from large-scale studies like that from Framingham, Massachusetts, also indicate that high blood levels of cholesterol increase the risk of a heart attack. In addition, there is a correlation between the amount of fat *in our diet* and the chances of a heart attack.

What Is Cholesterol?

Cholesterol is a waxy substance that is necessary for numerous body functions, especially the production of sex hormones and various body cells. Dietary and blood cholesterol are two different things. *Dietary* cholesterol is found in food of animal origin. *Blood* cholesterol is a measurement of the amount of this substance circulating in the bloodstream. It is measured in milligrams (1/1000 of a gram) per deciliter (100 cc, or about 1/10 of a quart or liter)—for example, 250 mg/dl. Dietary cholesterol is *only* found in food from animals, that is, meats, dairy products such as milk and cheese, and eggs. *Fruits, grains, and vegetables contain no cholesterol.* Messages on food packages like "cholesterol-free potato chips" are misleading when they imply that cholesterol has been removed. Potato chips never contained any cholesterol in the first place. It is also misleading to suggest that a "no-cholesterol food" is always a healthy food. It may be, but many foods free of cholesterol are high in fat and may present more of a problem than a cholesterol-containing, less fatty food. Good examples are some of the breakfast cereals with "no cholesterol" but a fair amount of saturated fat in the form of coconut oil, or those potato chips that are "cholesterol-free" but contain quite a bit of fat. Don't be misled by this type of labeling. Other examples of misleading labeling include items like nondairy creamer, advertised as being 100 percent cholesterol-free—it is, but 100 percent of its calories come from fat. Bologna or beef franks, advertised as containing "25 to 30 percent less fat" may be less fatty than before, but more than 50 percent of their calories still come from fat.

Most of the cholesterol in the body is derived from saturated fat. The new FDA regulations should help clarify the problem of misleading statements. Read the labels; they list *exactly* how much fat (saturated and total) and cholesterol are contained in each food. Each of our recipes lists total calories, fat grams, and the amount of cholesterol in a serving. For example, Larry Forgione's recipe for Steamed Mussels with Fennel in an Orange Broth on page 171 contains 255 calories per serving, 9.4 g of total fat (84 calories as fat), 4 g of saturated fat (36 calories as saturated fat), and 124 mg of cholesterol.

Measuring Cholesterol—The Good and the Bad

Recent emphasis on the several types of cholesterol in the blood has at least partially clarified the issue of why some people with total blood cholesterol levels considered to be within the normal range still develop heart disease. Although there are many cholesterol subfractions there are two major ones: 1) high-density lipoproteins, or HDL, the so-called good cholesterol that actually helps remove excess cholesterol from the blood and thereby decreases the amount available for plaque formation; and 2) low-density lipoproteins, or LDL, the so-called bad cholesterol, which is the major component of the fatty material in atherosclerotic deposits in artery walls.

Cholesterol is carried in the bloodstream in combination with a protein covering or package as lipoproteins ("lipo" means fat). The lipoproteins include cholesterol and its fractions. The average blood cholesterol content in Americans is about 210 to 215 mg/dl. The ranges and classifications of total cholesterol and HDLs are summarized in Table 6. A total cholesterol level above 240 may appear to indicate an increased risk but the ratio of the amount of total cholesterol to HDL may be a more important indicator of risk than total cholesterol alone. A desirable ratio is about 4.5:1 or lower. Thus, a total cholesterol of 260 or 270 may not indicate an increased risk of a heart attack if the HDL is higher than 65 or 70 (260/65 = a ratio of 4.1). Women tend to have high HDL levels until about five to ten years after menopause. This may explain why heart attacks are relatively uncommon in women below the ages of fifty-five or sixty.

Table 6

CLASSIFICATION OF BLOOD CHOLESTEROL LEVELS*

	TOTAL CHOLESTEROL LEVEL	HIGH DENSITY LIPOPROTEIN (HDL)
LOW RISK	BELOW 200 (DESIRABLE)	ABOVE 45–50
MODERATE RISK	200–239 (BORDERLINE HIGH)	35–45
INCREASED RISK	240 (HIGH)†	BELOW 35

A ratio of total cholesterol to HDL higher than 4.5 indicates an increased risk for heart disease:

EXAMPLE: TOTAL CHOLESTEROL

$$\frac{250}{40} = 6.25 \text{ (INCREASED RISK)}$$

HDL CHOLESTEROL

On the other hand, a high cholesterol level of 275 does not imply an increased risk if the HDL level is 70 to 75.‡

$$\frac{275}{75} = 3.7 \text{ (LOW RISK)}$$

NOTE: *The higher the HDL level, the lower the risk for heart disease.*

Treatment decisions should be guided not only by lipid levels (cholesterol, HDL, and LDL) but by the presence or absence of other risk factors.

†*Even high levels of cholesterol in the blood may not pose a greatly increased risk of heart disease in someone without other risk factors or with a high HDL level.*

‡*This type of finding is not uncommon in premenopausal women, who often have high HDL levels (these often decrease as estrogen levels decrease after menopause).*

Generally, people stay on the same cholesterol track after ages thirty to forty. If your cholesterol level is low, that is, 180 to 200, at age thirty-five, it may increase to some degree at ages forty, fifty, and sixty, but unless you gain weight or dramatically change what you eat, it will probably not go into the 250 to 260 or 280 range.

What About LDL, or Low-Density Lipoprotein, Levels?

LDL levels generally follow along with total cholesterol levels—a high total cholesterol level usually indicates a high LDL level. So for purposes of simplicity, it is not unscientific to just think about total and HDL levels when considering whether you are at risk and what you should do about it (there are exceptions to this rule but not many). This is not exactly the way the guidelines from the National Heart, Lung and Blood Institute evaluate the cholesterol issue, but other countries have adopted this approach. If you are used to tracking your LDL levels, the guidelines in the following table might be helpful, but you probably don't have to get involved with these numbers.

TABLE 7

LDL LEVELS AND CLINICAL CONDITION

CLINICAL CONDITION	DESIRABLE LEVELS OF LDL (MG/DL)	MEDICAL THERAPY INDICATED LDL LEVELS (MG/DL)
I. WITHOUT HEART DISEASE AND FEWER THAN TWO OTHER RISK FACTORS FOR HEART DISEASE	BELOW 160	ABOVE 190
II. WITHOUT HEART DISEASE BUT WITH MORE THAN TWO RISK FACTORS FOR HEART DISEASE, I.E., HIGH BLOOD PRESSURE, SMOKER, DIABETES, ETC.	BELOW 130	ABOVE 160
III. KNOWN HEART DISEASE	BELOW 100–110	ABOVE 130

What About Triglycerides?

These are other fatty substances in the blood. Levels are increased in obesity and in subjects with diabetes. Alcohol consumption may increase triglyceride levels. To date, there is some but not conclusive evidence that an elevated level of triglycerides by itself is an independent risk factor for coronary heart disease. These components probably play some role in promoting atherosclerosis or increasing blood clotting. In other words, keeping the level of triglycerides in the blood below 250 is a good idea. Dietary and other interventions undertaken to lower total cholesterol (and LDL) levels or increase HDL levels will often lower triglyceride levels. Losing weight is the most effective triglyceride-lowering intervention. Eating fish with large amounts of a certain kind of unsaturated fatty oil (omega-3 oil) may also help to lower the level of triglycerides in the blood.

What Determines the Amount of Cholesterol in Your Blood

We all know people whose cholesterol levels increase if they so much as look at an egg. And we know other people who eat eggs, red meat, or dairy products whenever they wish and live long, healthy lives with normal cholesterol levels and no heart disease. These people are fortunate in having large numbers of chemical substances (receptors) in their livers that help rid their systems of the cholesterol they take in. Most of us fall somewhere between these two extremes. Actually, our livers (if normal), produce enough cholesterol for most of us to function quite well even if we drastically reduce both our fat and cholesterol intakes.

In this book, we show you how you can eat some foods containing fat and cholesterol, that is, meat, fish, shellfish, and dairy products, without having your cholesterol levels increase; in fact, if you follow our advice, these levels will decrease in many instances. As we have noted, and will *reemphasize* as we go over recipes and menus, that less than 25 percent of your total daily calories should be fat calories; less than 7 to 8 percent should be calories from saturated fat. Your total cholesterol intake should be less than 250 mg. These recommendations are only slightly different from the American Heart Association's Step 2 Diet and are not difficult to follow even as you enjoy gourmet cooking. As we have also stated, if you exceed these amounts one day, cut back or budget your intake for the next two or three days to maintain a balance. *If you fall into a very high risk category, especially if you have heart disease, you are better off limiting total and saturated fat intake still further (to below 20 and 7 to 8 percent, respectively)* and *cholesterol intake to below 200 mg/day.* Even this is not as difficult as you might think. Go ahead and enjoy Larry Forgione's Black Bean Salad with Grilled Chicken (page 94) for lunch, followed by Jimmy Schmidt's Nectarine and Blackberry Crisp (page 117). You've used up 1,058 calories, 25.4 g of total fat (229 calories), 7.6 g of saturated fat (68 calories) and 77.1 mg cholesterol. You're well under the 500 calories of fat suggested in the 2,000-calories/day diet. But for the rest of the day be careful, just have a usual breakfast of cereal and orange juice and a single serving (about a cup) of a pasta dish and fruit for dinner—not too bad, and you're still within your fairly rigid budget. Check the Two-Week Menu Plan and see how easily this is done.

What Is Your Personal Risk?

A careful explanation of how cholesterol levels in the blood affect someone's risk for heart disease may be out of place in a book about good food and healthy eating, but if you are interested in knowing what your risk really is, we discuss this in the Appendix of this book.

The bottom line is that 1) while elevated blood cholesterol levels are important, they should not be the only targets of any program to reduce the risk of atherosclerosis; and 2) young people (below fifty years of age) and especially women who are active, thin, nonsmokers, do not have diabetes or hypertension, and have no evidence of heart disease or an enlarged heart are not at great additional risk unless blood cholesterol levels are extremely high (above 290 to 300), or unless other fractions of blood fats are very abnormal. These are the people who may need specific therapy if dietary changes are not effective.

Many people have attempted to estimate how much longer someone might live if he or she reduced blood cholesterol from a high level of 250 to a more desirable level of 200 to 210. Depending on who does the calculation, life expectancy might be increased only by two to three or six to eight months, if the person is in a low-risk group. But it's a different story for people who are obese, have high blood pressure, or smoke, that is, those with other risk factors. It is even more important for people who already have evidence of heart disease to keep their blood cholesterol levels as low as possible.

Assess your risk of developing heart disease on the basis of these factors and then you can, along with your doctor or dietician, decide on what kind of a calorie- or fat-budget program is best for you. Obviously, if you're at high risk, your approach will be different than if you're at low risk.

Controlling Cholesterol

You can control your intake of dietary cholesterol by watching what you eat. Unfortunately this may or may not always affect the levels of blood cholesterol, but in most cases a low intake will reduce blood levels to some degree. Remember, though, that saturated fat intake is probably more important than cholesterol intake in determining blood cholesterol levels. Saturated fat limits the removal of cholesterol by the LDL receptors in the liver—more cholesterol accumulates in the blood. Monounsaturated fat like olive oil may be high in calories but does not increase the risk of a heart attack and may actually reduce LDL cholesterol levels in the blood.

DIETARY RECOMMENDATIONS FOR CONTROLLING CHOLESTEROL LEVELS

- Prepare meals with as little added fat as possible. Use small amounts of polyunsaturated or monosaturated margarine or oil for spreads and cooking.
- Place more emphasis on eating fresh fruit and vegetables and whole-grain products to achieve a lower intake of fat and a higher intake of fiber, vitamins C and E, and beta carotene.
- Include at least two servings each day of low-fat or skim milk products to ensure an adequate intake of calcium.
- Include fresh fish at least twice a week.
- Exclude dairy, meat, or hardened vegetable fats in cooking, spreads, and ingredients in home-baked products.
- Limit red meat (lean cuts) to less than 120 g (4 ounces) four to five days a week for men, and 90 g (3 ounces) for women. If regular cheese is used as a replacement for meat meals (30 g, or 1 ounce, of cheese replaces a portion of lean meat), this should be done no more than twice a week. (These recommendations may appear to be out of line for a low-fat diet, but as you will see, you can eat meat or cheese and still stay within the guidelines.)
- Restrict eggs to no more than two or three each week. Unlimited amounts of Egg Beaters (liquid egg substitute) and egg whites are acceptable.

Table 8 gives you an idea of some foods high in cholesterol; these should be avoided or eaten in small amounts. Or, if you binge on some shrimp one day, be more careful the next. Note that most of these foods (with the major exceptions of shellfish) also have a high fat content. Remember that a *4-ounce* serving of meat or poultry is just a little larger than the size of a deck of cards or the palm of a man's hand—most portions served in a restaurant are 6 to 8 ounces—you'll have to adjust for the extra calories if you indulge. *Sizes of portions do count.* Most books on nutrition list the contents of 3-ounce portions. We think that this is unrealistic because most people will probably eat larger quantities, no matter what is suggested. Some of our recipes call for 5- or 6-ounce servings of meat or fish, others call for 4-ounce servings. If you eat a smaller portion, adjust the numbers accordingly.

TABLE 8

FOODS WITH A HIGH CHOLESTEROL CONTENT*

FOOD (4 OZ.)	CHOLESTEROL† (MG)	SATURATED FAT (G)	TOTAL FAT (G)	TOTAL CALORIES
MEATS				
Beef				
Liver	546	3	9	245
Kidneys	438	1	4	163
Brisket, whole, lean only	111	7	21	284
Ground beef, lean	115	8	20	317
Lamb				
Leg, roasted	101	3	9	216
Pork				
Liverwurst	179	12	32	370
Spareribs, braised	137	13	34	450
Tenderloin‡	119	6	17	309
Loin pork chops‡	119	6	17	309
Veal				
Cutlet, braised	134	8	20	322
Poultry				
Egg (1 whole)	212	2	5	78
Turkey, dark meat without skin	96	3	8	211
Chicken, dark meat without skin	108	4	12	236
Chicken, light meat without skin	96	1	4	186
Seafood				
Shrimp, steamed	221	0.3	1	112
Crab, blue, steamed	113	0.3	2	114

FOODS WITH MODERATE AMOUNTS OF CHOLESTEROL BUT LOW LEVELS OF TOTAL AND SATURATED FAT

Mackerel, broiled	68	3	12	228
Lobster, steamed	81	0.1	1	111
Cod, broiled	53	0.1	1	119
Swordfish	57	2	6	175
Halibut, broiled	47	0.5	3	159

FOODS WITH MODERATE AMOUNTS OF CHOLESTEROL
AND A HIGH FAT CONTENT

FOOD (4 OZ.)	CHOLESTEROL† (MG)	SATURATED FAT (G)	TOTAL FAT (G)	TOTAL CALORIES
Hot dogs (2)	69	14	32	358
Italian sausage	89	10	29	366

Some of these foods may also contain a high content of fat.

†Total intake of cholesterol should not exceed 250 mg/day.

‡Despite what most people think, there are many cuts of pork that are relatively low in total and saturated fat and calories. For example, 4 ounces of ham has only 2 g of saturated fat, 6 g of total fat, and 175 calories. Many pork dishes are okay in a fat-budget program, but watch out for spareribs and sausages.

When using this table, keep several things in mind: 1) Total cholesterol intake in food should not exceed 250 mg/day (the lower the better); 2) total fat intake should not exceed 25 percent of total calories (each gram of fat = 9 calories, more than twice the number of calories as a gram of protein or carbohydrate). On a 2,000-calorie/day intake a maximum of 500 calories should come from fat (500 divided by 9 = about 55 g/day). Two hot dogs or 4 ounces of Italian sausage use up a large percentage of the daily fat allowance. In our fat-budget diet, we actually keep the total fat calories below 25 percent.

Remember also to keep saturated fat below 7 to 8 percent of calories. On a 2,000-calorie/day diet, saturated fat should make up less than 200 calories, or about 22 g. Look at the difference between the saturated fat content of a frankfurter or liverwurst and most fish and poultry (without skin). No one is going to be counting the contents of every morsel of food—*nor do they have to*—but getting a general idea of the worst offenders (that is, foods highest in saturated fat) is helpful. And once you do it, it's done.

Blood cholesterol levels may in some instances be reduced by exercise. Active people, especially those who engage in moderate exercise three or four times a week, also tend to have higher HDL ("good" cholesterol) levels than sedentary people. As noted, premenopausal women, who still produce large amounts of estrogen, also tend to have high levels of HDL; their HDL levels might be 70, 80, or even 90 (a normal range is approximately 50 to 55). That's one of the reasons why women in their thirties and forties with cholesterol levels of 260, 270, or even 300 are not necessarily at great risk for heart disease; their total cholesterol to HDL ratio is less than 4.5:1.

Keeping thin is another good way to control blood cholesterol. Obese people tend to have higher cholesterol levels *and* lower HDL levels than thin, active people.

When and How Often to Test for Cholesterol

Every adult over the age of twenty should have his or her blood cholesterol level measured. This is especially important if there is a family history of early onset of heart disease—this means heart disease in parents or siblings before the age of fifty-five or sixty. If cholesterol levels are normal (200 or below), there is no reason to test them more than about every three or four years.

We do not believe that it is necessary to routinely test children for cholesterol levels. This suggestion is in contrast to recent recommendations of several national medical organizations that suggest routine tests at age two or three. Exceptions should be made for children from families with strong histories of premature heart disease or exceptionally high fat levels in the blood. In general, screening children may produce unwarranted anxiety in parents. Since we should be encouraging healthful eating habits and plenty of exercise for our offspring anyway, we probably wouldn't change anything if cholesterol levels were shown to be above a certain level. Drugs are rarely indicated in children unless they fall into an unusual category—selective testing of a small percentage of children at high risk is probably appropriate.

Review Table 6 for our interpretations of the cholesterol levels that we believe should be cause for concern and careful monitoring. Keep in mind that cholesterol levels should never be viewed in a vacuum. If they are elevated and no other risk factors are present, risk associated with the elevations may not be great enough to warrant anything other than a modification of diet.

CHOLESTEROL LEVELS: WHO IS AT RISK?

Elevated blood cholesterol levels predict heart disease risk. Keep cholesterol below 240 mg/dl, if possible. Young women without other risk factors who tend to have elevated levels of high-density lipoproteins and the elderly (age seventy to seventy-five or older) *without other risk factors* or heart disease probably need not pay as close attention to cholesterol levels as the rest of the population. If there is any question about your risk factor status or what to do about an elevated cholesterol level, you should consult your doctor.

Lowering Cholesterol Levels

To answer the questions of whether blood, or serum, cholesterol levels can be reduced by diet and whether HDL cholesterols can be increased by increased physical activity, it is necessary to look at the success rates of people who have followed the American Heart Association's Step 1 Diet. This diet suggests no more than 30 percent of total calorie intake should be total fat and no more than 10 percent of the total should be saturated fat. In addition, no more than 300 mg of cholesterol should be consumed daily. This is the diet recommended for people at otherwise low risk with moderately elevated cholesterol levels (about 240–260). In our experience even strict adherence to these recommendations has only lowered cholesterol levels by about 5 to 7 percent in most people (and to a lesser degree in some). In other words, if your cholesterol level was 250 to begin with, it might drop to about 230 to 235 after about three to six months on this Step 1 Diet.

The American Heart Association's Step 2 Diet keeps total fat at 30 percent of total calories, but suggests a reduction of saturated fat to less than 7 percent, and cholesterol intake to below 200 mg. This diet results in a more significant reduction of blood cholesterol and, as we will show you, *this level of intake is not too difficult for most people to achieve and is similar but not exactly the same as the one that we advocate in the book.*

Several studies have demonstrated that a reduction of blood cholesterol levels of about

10 plus percent has reduced the incidence of recurrent heart attacks in people with known heart disease.

One of the most effective ways to reduce blood cholesterol is to lose weight. Even being 5 to 10 pounds overweight (see A Simple Method to Figure Your Ideal Weight (page 11) can raise your cholesterol levels; if you lose even these 5 to 10 pounds, you may notice a decrease in cholesterol levels. If you are truly overweight or obese and lose 15, 20, or more pounds, the drop will be more significant. To keep your heart attack risk as low as possible, it is equally or perhaps even more important to stop smoking and to maintain a normal blood pressure.

What About Exercise and Cholesterol Levels?

There is some evidence that a moderate degree of exercise over time will help to increase HDL levels. This is not a universal finding, however, but since exercise helps to burn calories and makes you feel better, this is clearly something that everyone should pursue. Increasing your level of activity is important, and no one can argue that strenuous exercise may be a good way to keep your weight down and your body fit. But it is not the answer for everyone. In fact, lots of people have been discouraged from starting any exercise program because they have been told that only the vigorous kind is beneficial. Years ago we pointed out that heart attack risk can be reduced and weight loss aided by moderate, enjoyable, non-ankle-, hip- or knee-stressing exercises. This advice is still appropriate, notwithstanding, a recent study that emphasized the benefits of strenuous exercise. Moderate exercise, even walking or relaxed bike riding, is a good way to help take off weight and to keep it off once lost—and possibly to reduce cholesterol levels. Walking at a 2- to 3-mile-per-hour pace for thirty to forty-five minutes three to four times a week may be just as beneficial as more vigorous and "harder to follow through" (or maintain enthusiasm for) programs.

Table 1 (page 15) will give you an idea of just how many calories are burned up with various activities. Without some calorie reduction, exercise alone will not usually result in weight loss or a definite change in cholesterol levels. Playing tennis may burn about 300 to 400 calories an hour, but few of us have ten hours a week, week after week, to devote to tennis so that we can lose a pound or two. (Remember: to lose 1 pound you must burn up about 3,500 more calories than you take in.)

What to Expect

If you were able to stay on a vegetarian diet and, if overweight, adhere to a rigid weight-loss program that resulted in a significant loss of 20 to 30 pounds, then a decrease of 20 to 30 percent in serum (blood) cholesterol and LDL levels might occur. Some people are able to lose weight and keep it off with this type of regimen, *but most are not*. The majority of people also do not enjoy or tolerate a vegetarian diet for other than short periods of time. Rather than give up meat and poultry completely, we propose a compromise that includes lots of vegetables and grains but fish, meat, and poultry, too.

If our *less rigid but enjoyable* approach to keeping healthy helps keep cholesterol levels within a satisfactory range, great, but if it does not, it may be a better idea to take some medication if you are in the moderate- or high-risk category. This may sound like strange advice in a book about good nutrition and enjoyable eating, but it may be good advice and has been successfully pursued in several heart studies and with my own patients. The most important thing to remember is not to take medication if you are *not* truly at risk. The situation with high blood pressure provides a good analogy to this. If a reasonable diet and exercise program doesn't work, medication is advisable. Probably more than one third of hypertensive patients could have their blood pressures reduced to normal *if* a *rigid* low-salt and low-calorie diet were followed, but this is impractical for most of us. There are some people with less severe hypertension whose blood pressures will decrease to normal levels with a lesser degree of salt restriction, and a weight loss and exercise program that they, as individuals, are able to follow. But, most of the time, this will not be successful. About 70 to 80 percent of people with high blood pressure will have to take some medication to keep their pressure normal in an effort to prevent heart, brain, and kidney disease. So, if the program we suggest in this book doesn't lower your cholesterol or blood pressure and your doctor determines that you are one of those people at higher risk, you probably should take some medication.

In persons with evidence of heart disease, whether they have angina or have had a heart attack, it is extremely important to reduce cholesterol levels to as low as possible. In these cases, a target level of below 180 to 200 is justified. Regression or shrinkage of some of the lesions in the coronary arteries may occur if this can be accomplished.

SOME MEDICATIONS USED TO REDUCE BLOOD CHOLESTEROL LEVELS

Nicotinic acid (niacin) is a vitamin that, when used in dosages of 1,000 to 3,000 mg/day (1 to 3g), will reduce total cholesterol, LDL, and triglyceride levels while increasing the HDL content of the blood. In some ways, it is an ideal blood-fat-lowering medication. But in dosages necessary to produce a definite effect, niacin often causes side effects such as flushing, headaches, and palpitations that many people can't tolerate. Building up to an effective dosage slowly and taking dosages with food will help reduce side effects. So will taking an aspirin a day, which is a good idea anyway since it has been demonstrated in numerous studies that even a baby aspirin a day helps to prevent heart attacks by reducing the tendency of the blood to clot. Newer, more slowly absorbed formulations of niacin may cause fewer side effects but may cause other problems. Large doses of niacin may precipitate gout or adversely affect sugar metabolism.

Newer drugs, such as *lovastatin (Mevacor), simvastatin (Zocor),* and *pravastatin (Pravachol),* are highly effective, decreasing LDL and total cholesterol levels by 20–35 percent. They are easy to take and generally safe. Blood chemistries should be monitored periodically to detect liver function changes that may occur with these drugs. Severe muscle pain may also be seen in a very few people. These are medications that we have used with good results. Recent studies have demonstrated a slowing down of the process of atherosclerosis when these are given. *Gemfibrozil* or *probucol* may be indicated for some people.

Estrogen replacement therapy in postmenopausal women may raise HDL and decrease LDL and total cholesterol levels.

Medications to Lower Cholesterol Levels

Hopefully, our program of a prudent, easy-to-follow diet and regular exercise will keep your cholesterol levels within a reasonable range. But there are quite a few people who require drug therapy. Fortunately, there are many choices of reasonably safe drugs that work (see Medications Used to Reduce Blood Cholesterol Levels). Some of the medications suggested by the National Cholesterol Committee, of the National Heart, Lung and Blood Institute specifically *cholestyramine* and *colestipol*, may lower cholesterol levels in the blood but are difficult for most people to take. These medications bind cholesterol and fatty acids in the intestinal tract and help the body excrete rather than absorb them. The drugs frequently cause uncomfortable bloating and numerous gastrointestinal symptoms. So, while effective, they may not be the medications of choice and we do not often prescribe them.

Heart Disease and "Hardening of the Arteries"

T he term "hardening of the arteries" has been used for generations to explain some of the changes that occur in the walls of arteries as we age. Arteries do not actually harden but become less elastic and develop certain characteristics that may result in heart and blood vessel disease. At birth, the inside linings of the arteries—the blood vessels that supply blood to tissues—are perfectly smooth; blood flows easily through them. As we get older, deposits of fatty materials (which contain cholesterol) and various cells begin to build up within the walls of the arteries. These collections are called "plaque." As the plaque thickens or enlarges, it narrows the opening in the arteries through which blood travels to various muscles and organs. The medical term for this process is *atherosclerosis*.

The consequences of hardening or narrowing of the arteries may be quite serious. If one of the coronary arteries, which supply blood to the heart muscle, narrows or closes off, certain parts of the muscle are deprived of blood—and a heart attack occurs. A stroke results when one of the arteries carrying blood to a portion of the brain closes off. Everything we talk about when we discuss reducing our risk of heart or blood vessel disease relates to slowing down the process of plaque formation in arteries.

The Causes of Hardening of the Arteries (Atherosclerosis)

Medical science has devoted years to studying the processes that initiate or increase atherosclerosis. Epidemiologists, the detectives of medicine, have determined that certain factors speed the process. Some of these we cannot do anything about: aging, heredity, or being male, which increases the risk of atherosclerosis at an earlier age than for females. But some of the most important risk factors *can* be influenced by either behavioral changes, diet, or medication. Obesity, diabetes, an elevated blood cholesterol level, high blood pressure, smoking, and a sedentary life-style are all risks that can be reduced.

The process of atherosclerosis is considered a progressive one and is, as expected, most extensive among the elderly. Certain population groups, however, appear to have less hardening of the arteries than others. The French, Japanese, and Italians and many primitive societies, for example, are less apt to develop the problem. The intake of saturated fat is low in these populations. Thus, there are older people in these groups whose arteries remain relatively free of plaque formation. In the United States, studies have shown that the coronary arteries (arteries that supply blood to the heart muscle) in some young men aged eighteen to twenty-five who were killed in accidents or wars already had some evidence of plaque formation. This strongly suggests that for many of us, at least in our society and especially in men, prevention should start early—and starting early means paying attention to risk factors—and to *the type of foods we eat*.

Anyone with a strong *family history* of heart disease, particularly those with parents who developed heart disease before the age of fifty-five to sixty, are at a greater risk of developing atherosclerosis at a younger age than other people. The process is not inevitable, however, and can be delayed to a considerable extent by doing what we're describing in this book—keeping controllable risk factors in check—without necessarily depriving yourself of the enjoyable things in life.

Smoking may be the most important risk factor for speeding up the process of hardening of the arteries. Evidence indicates that it is *not* the nicotine that causes damage to blood vessels; the smoke or carbon monoxide and some chemical particles in tobacco smoke injure the smooth lining of the artery wall and enable fatty material to seep into the wall and build up under the surface. Smoking is something to avoid, whether there is a family history of heart disease or not. Some people feel safe when they smoke filtered cigarettes, but they are fooling themselves. While these may contain less nicotine and tars and may therefore be less damaging to lung tissue, the amount of carbon monoxide inhaled may actually be greater with a filtered cigarette than with an unfiltered one. Data suggest that blood vessel damage may be increased, not decreased, when a low-nicotine cigarette is used. Nicotine intake does transiently increase heart rate and may raise blood pressure levels but it is probably not the ingredient in a cigarette that speeds up atherosclerosis.

The message here is easy: Don't smoke if you want to reduce your heart, vascular, and lung disease risk. Fortunately, millions of people have heeded the message. The percentage of smokers in the United States has decreased in all population groups except among young women. Cigar or pipe smoking do not increase the risk of heart disease, since very little smoke is inhaled. However, the incidence of cancer of the lip and tongue increases in these smokers. Chewing tobacco is also not a good idea if you want to avoid cancer of the mouth.

As previously noted, *high levels of cholesterol* in the blood have also been identified as a major risk factor for premature hardening of the arteries. If the lining of your blood vessels has been damaged by smoking or high blood pressure and your blood fat (cholesterol) levels are high, there is an increased risk of the extra fat collecting beneath the lining of the vessel and increasing the degree of plaque formation. If you have a low blood cholesterol level, there will be less of a chance of developing atherosclerosis, even if you have high blood pressure and damaged blood vessel linings.

In the previous chapter regarding cholesterol, the discussion of its components—the "good" HDLs and the "bad" LDLs—hopefully has clarified some of the confusing misinformation that has produced unnecessary anxiety in thousands of people.

The third very important major risk factor for heart disease and strokes is *high blood pressure* (the medical term for which is *hypertension*). A previous book of mine, *Lower Your Blood Pressure and Live Longer* (Berkley Books, 1991, in paperback) discusses high blood pressure in detail. This can be referred to for more information, but some basic facts are important to understand. Keeping your weight down, exercising, and staying on a low-fat, low-cholesterol diet will not do you as much good as it should if you continue to walk around with elevated blood pressure. High blood pressure damages the endothelium (inner lining) of arteries. This accelerates atherosclerosis. If your blood pressure is lowered to normal, the process can be arrested or perhaps reversed.

Normal blood pressure ranges from about 110/80 to 135 to 140/85 to 90 (see Table 9: Blood Pressure Categories). Contrary to what most people believe, blood pressure is highest in the early morning just before or as we awaken between approximately six-thirty and eight A.M. This may be one reason that heart attacks are more common in the morning. Pressure is lowest between one and six A.M. when we sleep. Also, contrary to common belief, the systolic blood pressure (upper reading) may be more important in estimating heart disease risk than the bottom or lower reading, the diastolic pressure. If your blood pressure is consistently higher than 140/90 (regardless of your age) on repeated measurements, you have hypertension and should be treated. This does not necessarily mean that you have to take medication; your blood pressure may be controllable through diet and exercise.

It is important to note that so-called white-coat hypertension—that is, blood pressures that are high in a doctor's office but normal at home—should be treated and not ignored. People with this type of variable blood pressure may already have early changes in the walls of arteries or in heart muscle. These changes usually become more marked if the pressure is not controlled.

TABLE 9
BLOOD PRESSURE CATEGORIES FOR ADULTS*

	SYSTOLIC (MM HG)	DIASTOLIC (MM HG)
Normal	below 130–135	85 or below
High normal	135–139	85–89
High		
Stage 1 (mild)	140–159	90–99
Stage 2 (moderately severe)	160–179	100–109
Stage 3 (severe)	180–209	110–119
Stage 4 (very severe)	higher than 210	120 or higher

Blood pressure is recorded as 120 (systolic—recorded when the heart is pumping) over 80 (diastolic—recorded when the heart is resting between beats), or 120/80. Several readings are usually taken and the numbers averaged. Blood pressure may vary by 15 to 20 mm Hg during the day.

What Causes High Blood Pressure?

In about 90 percent of cases of hypertension, we are not absolutely certain what causes it. We do know that blood pressure goes up because certain blood vessels constrict or narrow. Think of a pump and a hose with a nozzle—if the pump is working and the nozzle is partially closed, the pressure of water in the tubing will be higher than if the nozzle is wide open. We have some clues as to why the arteries that regulate blood pressure constrict more easily in some people than in others. Genetic differences most likely play a role in causing this to occur and in causing high blood pressure. Anyone with a strong family history of hypertension tends to develop it more readily than someone whose close relations all have normal blood pressure.

Some people are "salt sensitive": a high intake of salt increases their blood pressure; reducing salt lowers it. In others, salt intake does not appear to be important. There is good evidence to indicate that in populations that consume large amounts of salt (that is, more than 10 g or about 2 teaspoons of salt, which equals 4 g of sodium a day) blood pressures are generally higher. It is the mineral sodium, a component of salt, that contributes to accumulation of excess fluid and elevated blood pressure. We will point out the sodium content in the recipes in this book so that if you are put on a low-sodium diet by your doctor to control your blood pressure or fluid accumulation you will know which recipes to modify, use sparingly, or, in some instances, avoid completely. (Low-sodium diets usually imply an intake of less than 2 g, or 2,000 mg, of sodium a day. Most of our recipes contain relatively small amounts of sodium. Some, however, like Jimmy Schmidt's Vegetable Black Bean Chili on page 162, contain just too much sodium (842 mg per serving) for someone who is supposed to limit his or her intake to less than 2,000 mg a day.

In a few incidences (about 4 to 5 percent of cases) kidney disease or narrowing of one of the arteries to one of the kidneys results in high blood pressure. In less than a half of one percent of cases, blood pressure is elevated because of specific tumors in the glands that secrete adrenaline or certain hormones and are located on top of each kidney. In these few instances, surgery can cure hypertension.

As troubling as it may be to the patient and his doctor not to be able to pinpoint the exact cause of high blood pressure, this need not affect treatment in most cases. Luckily, treatment is highly effective today. In the 1940s and early 1950s, many thousands of people with high blood pressure progressed to heart and kidney failure or had strokes or heart attacks. Today, these complications are far less common. Modern therapy has dramatically reduced strokes and stroke deaths, heart failure, and heart attacks. Importantly, treatment need not involve hospitalizations or expensive or complicated regimens.

No one knows the exact number, but about 20 to 25 percent of people with high blood pressure may be able to reduce pressures to normal simply by losing weight, exercising more, and reducing salt intake. If you are one of these, you should be able to do this without becoming involved in unpleasant, rigid, or expensive kinds of dieting programs. Eventually, however, most patients with hypertension will have to take some medication.

If you are put on medication, don't be upset or discouraged. There are numerous effective medications available so that almost anyone, even those people with severe hypertension, should be able to have his or her pressures reduced to normal levels. A large majority will tolerate medication without any side effects.

It is important to keep the risk factors for heart disease and hardening of the arteries in mind as we discuss methods to reduce them and show you how a major part of the problem—eating the wrong foods—can be changed in a pleasant, enjoyable way without deprivation.

ABOUT THE CHEFS AND THE RECIPES

Three of the country's leading chefs contributed the recipes for this book. Working independently of each other, they created dishes for breakfast, lunch, and dinner, concentrating on making each one relatively low in fat and calories but high in flavor and culinary inspiration. However, none of the chefs has jumped on the low-fat bandwagon that so often defines the cooking of the nineties. They simply strive to serve excellent food prepared with the utmost integrity and care. The recipes that follow reflect this philosophy, while underlining our premise that foods that are *extremely* low in fat and cholesterol are not necessary for "healthy eating." While their styles of cooking differ one from the other, all three chefs have been praised for ingenuity and creativity. And just as importantly, each in his or her own way, has contributed significantly to the elevation of American cuisine.

All cook with the freshest ingredients and believe that using those foods that are in season is ultimately satisfying, not to mention efficient in terms of cost and availability. Alice Waters, on the West Coast, has access to locally grown produce nearly all year long. Jimmy Schmidt, in Detroit, and Larry Forgione, in New York City, rely on local produce too, but because they face long winters, they must turn at times to other parts of the country for their ingredients.

"Foods in season taste the best," says Jimmy Schmidt from The Rattlesnake Club, his award-winning Detroit, Michigan, restaurant. "My focus is entirely on flavor. Overall my tastes have been directed away from meat and fish and toward utilizing the natural flavors of seasonal ingredients."

Echoing this, Alice Waters, owner of the renowned Chez Panisse in Berkeley, California, suggests that foods used in season require very little preparation. "If you buy ripe tomatoes in the height of summer, dinner is ready!" she says. "As we [at the restaurant] learned as we became more involved in our garden, you can cut the amount of salt in half and often need no sugar at all when the produce is fresh and in season. This is very different from when we began twenty years ago. Then, we added salt, sugar, butter, and oil to food to make it rich."

At An American Place, Larry Forgione's three-star restaurant in the heart of New York City, less reliance on animal protein, fats, and oils is common practice today. In fact, red meat never appears on the lunch menu, although it is always on the dinner menu.

"From what I have read, the number one concern about the American diet is the volume of fat we consume," says the chef. "But it is hard to eliminate fat in your diet because its absence often means flavors are flat. When I reduce fat, I look for other ingredients to compensate, because I will not sacrifice flavor."

When developing the recipes that appear on the following pages, Larry explained that he began with an idea that he knew would taste good. "From there, I worked backward to eliminate fats while balancing the flavors with ingredients that enhanced the overall flavor profile of the dish." He used small quantities of high-quality olive oil and bolstered the flavor with ingredients such as ginger, garlic, fresh herbs, spices, drained capers, low-fat stocks, and vinegar. He also used foods high in complex carbohydrates but low in fat, such as grains, pasta, and vegetables.

Jimmy and Alice essentially followed the same procedure. "As I became more knowledgeable, I learned how to balance good taste with good nutrition without having to give up flavor," reflects Jimmy. "This balance is crucial. For instance, while working on the recipes for this book we noticed a major change in our use of olive oil. We used to ladle the oil into the pans—common practice in restaurant kitchens—but now we use misters to spray a film of oil over the pan. The benefit is that our cooking is cleaner now, as well as lower in fat.

ANTIOXIDANT VITAMINS

Certain vitamins and other substances may prevent the low-density lipoproteins (LDL cholesterol) from becoming "oxidized," i.e., picking up extra oxygen in the blood that is left over from normal metabolism. Recipes that contain large amounts of these substances are noted.

Oxidized LDL initiates the process of atherosclerosis. Vitamins C, E and A appear to limit this process of oxidation. Some studies, especially with large doses of vitamin E, indicate that this may reduce heart attack risk.

Recommended Daily Allowances for Adults

Vitamin E: 8 mg for women, or about 12 international units (IU); 10 mg for men, or about 15 IU. (Vitamin E pills are available as 100, 200, and 400 units. These are equivalent to 65, 130, and 260 mg. Most studies on this vitamin are based on the use of these high-dose supplements.)

Vitamin C: 60 mg.

Beta Carotene: The body converts beta carotene to vitamin A. About 15 mg of beta carotene is equivalent to about 25,000 IU of vitamin A. About 4,000 IU of vitamin A are recommended daily for women and about 5,000 IU for men.

"The oven is very important, too," he continues. "You don't have to stir-fry or sauté everything in fat. Oven roasting and other slow-cooking techniques, which require very little fat, if any, allow foods such as vegetables to caramelize and take advantage of their natural sugars, which broadens the flavor of the dish."

Alice's style of cooking is described as Mediterranean, and she explains that a lot more olive oil is consumed in her kitchen than butter—a noticeable change from years earlier. At Chez Panisse, meat has almost been relegated to second-class status, usually showing up on the plates in 4-ounce portions, which is far less than most restaurant offerings.

"It has to do with moderation," Alice explains. "I eat a lot less meat than I used to and so do our customers." But her use of fresh vegetables, fruits, and herbs is never moderate, and as an outspoken champion of organic produce, she has led a nationwide crusade to encourage all Americans to seek out organically grown fruits and vegetables and organically raised poultry and meat.

Cooking with what is in season is Alice's passion. She happily anticipates June's peaches, July's fresh shell beans, August's tomatoes, and September's figs. Come winter, she looks forward to California's crop of greens: kale, chard, escarole, and mustard. Springtime brings asparagus, peas, and onions.

How the Recipes Are Arranged

Alice is not alone in her devotion to seasonal foods. Larry and Jimmy share the passion, and because of this, we have arranged the recipes in the book to reflect the seasons. We have also arranged them into meals, beginning with breakfast, continuing through lunch, and finishing with dinner—a meal that includes an appetizer and dessert. However, the imaginative reader will quickly determine, for instance, that some appetizers make lovely lunch dishes, and some lunch dishes are just right for supper. Also, these are not complete menus—they are groups of recipes that home cooks can integrate into their monthly menu plans. None is very high in fat, calories, or cholesterol and every one is full of flavor. The idea is that you can eat foods that taste good and are also good for you—and if you occasionally go overboard and consume more than your daily quota of calories and fat, nothing terrible will happen—if you remember the concept of fat budgeting.

Ingredients and Techniques

Chefs never tread the straight and narrow when it comes to recipes, and professionals as creative as Larry, Jimmy, and Alice avail themselves of a wide variety of foods. Because of this, some ingredients in some recipes may be unfamiliar to the home cook. We provide substitutions, buying information, or both, when an ingredient may be considered esoteric or hard to find—but we also encourage the home cook to stretch his or her culinary horizons in order to enjoy healthful eating while trying something new.

Throughout the book, the reader will find practical suggestions that render the more challenging recipes accessible to the home kitchen. For example, many recipes call for stocks. We provide recipes for these but, when appropriate, also suggest using canned broths or low-sodium bouillon cubes, if necessary. However, all three chefs encourage readers to make their own stock—and Alice in particular stresses how strongly she feels about this, saying she *never* relies on canned products: the "real" thing is so much better.

At times, the stock or another liquid is reduced, which means it is cooked for a period of time so that the water evaporates and leaves behind a slightly thickened, intensely flavored liquid. This classic technique may sound complicated, but it is not. It merely requires a little time. Straining a sauce is equally easy, although it may sound fussy to a novice. By the same token, many recipes are for grilling, but we always suggest broiling as an alternative to firing up the outside grill. Both cooking methods eliminate the need for fat.

All three chefs consider flavor tantamount, which makes preparing and serving these dishes a pleasure. As Jimmy Schmidt says, "It's not just nutrition; it's nourishment. Food is not simply 'fuel,' it's part of the fabric of life that makes it all worthwhile."

About the Nutritional Analysis

Following each recipe, we provide a nutritional analysis of the food to help readers plan a healthful diet while adhering to the fat budgeting concept. The analysis presents an approximate estimate of the calories, total fat, saturated fat, cholesterol, and sodium. In addition, we highlight those recipes that are high in fiber and certain vitamins. With fiber content, for example, we note that anything containing under 2 grams is relatively low in fiber, between

GARLIC

You will note that many of the recipes use garlic. (Those people who are sensitive to garlic and might develop abdominal cramps and diarrhea should adjust the recipes accordingly.) This adds flavor, but there is also some evidence that eating garlic may have a favorable effect on cholesterol levels. In addition, garlic may decrease the ability of the blood to clot—which, at least theoretically, could reduce the risk of heart attack. In a recent study we were unable to confirm these beneficial effects. More information is needed.

2 and 4 grams is a moderate source, between 4 and 6 grams is a good source and anything above 6 grams is a high or excellent source of fiber. For sodium content, any foods containing about 500 mg or more per serving should be considered high in sodium. Since many ingredients, such as chicken breasts, fruits, vegetables, fish fillets, and so on, vary significantly in size and because every cook's methods vary somewhat, your serving may contain slightly more or less of these values and nutrients.

NOTE: All recipes were analyzed using Food Processor Plus, version 5.03. The number of calories and the amounts of other ingredients listed are for the first food listed when a choice is given (eg. orange juice *or* cantaloupe).

When we analyzed the recipes we considered the following:

• All meats are trimmed of fat.
• Poultry skin is removed after cooking (unless the recipe specifies removing it before cooking).
• The size of the meat, poultry, and fish is calculated based on the cooked amount actually consumed.
• If a garnish or optional ingredient is included in the analysis, it is stated. Otherwise it is not included.
• The recipes that contain large amounts of vitamins C, E, and A are noted. These vitamins are singled out because they may have beneficial antioxidant properties that may help prevent heart disease. (Antioxidants may prevent LDL cholesterol from being deposited in the walls of arteries.) We make no claims that eating these preparations will supply enough antioxidants to do this, but we note their presence so that our readers will be aware of which foods are good sources of these nutrients.
• Although there is no Recommended Dietary Allowance for fiber, most health authorities recommend between 20 and 35 g a day for adults. There is some evidence that a high fiber intake may lower blood cholesterol levels and may reduce the risk of certain types of bowel cancer. *High fiber recipes are noted*.

FISH OILS AND FISH

Eating fish three to four times a week (at least) is good for you because fish is low in saturated fat and is a good source of protein. We have included a number of tasty fish recipes to supplement the tuna fish sandwiches that many people have for lunch. Go easy on the mayonaise if you make a tuna salad.

Many types of fish contain a great deal of polyunsaturated fat as oils called omega-3 oils. High intakes of these may reduce the tendency of blood to clot and may reduce blood fat content—factors that may help to prevent heart attack.

Low-fat fish include cod, flounder, grouper, sea bass, snapper, tuna, sea trout, and halibut.

Higher-fat or oily fish include swordfish, salmon, mackerel, herring, and blue fish. These fish have more fat than others but much of it is unsaturated fat and contains omega-3 oils.

Fish oil capsules contain omega-3 oils. To derive any benefit from these, you must take six to ten capsules a day. We advocate eating and enjoying fish rather than swallowing pills.

SPRING
RECIPES

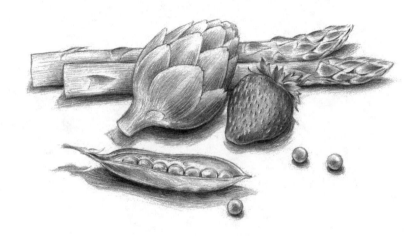

Breakfast

ALICE WATERS
....

COMPOTE OF TANGERINES AND BLOOD ORANGES

Serves 4

When blood oranges are in season—which is only briefly—Alice teams them with early spring tangerines and pale pink grapefruit for a jewel-toned compote sweetened only by the fruit itself. Blood oranges are grown in small numbers in California, and while the crop increases with demand, most varieties are imported to the United States from midwinter through midspring. They are smaller than most domestic oranges and, when cut open, yield deep red to almost purple flesh that is sublimely juicy and delicious.

3 tangerines
3 blood oranges
1 pink grapefruit
Juice of 1 additional grapefruit

Using a small sharp knife, gently peel the tangerine, oranges, and grapefruit to the flesh. Remove all white pith and strings. Carefully divide each into segments by inserting the knife between each segment and cutting sharply around the flesh at the fruit's core and coming back up the other side along the membrane. Hold the fruit over a small bowl to catch any juice. Drop the segments into the bowl as you separate them.

Pour the additional grapefruit juice over the fruit. Toss gently. Let stand for about 5 minutes before serving.

Nutritional Analysis per serving

Calories: 108
High in vitamin C
Fat: 0.4 g
Saturated Fat: 0 g
Cholesterol: 0 mg
Sodium: 1 mg
Relatively low source of fiber

JIMMY SCHMIDT
....

RAGOUT OF CITRUS WITH MAPLE SUGAR CRISPS

Serves 4

Grapefruit are at their best in the winter and springtime. This recipe calls for wonderfully sweet ruby red grapefruit from Texas and white grapefruit—the best coming from Florida's Indian River area. The low-fat breakfast is sweetened with maple sugar, which can be purchased from maple syrup suppliers and specialty shops. If need be, you can make a rough approximation by mixing equal measures of white granulated and light brown sugar.

2 large white grapefruit
2 large ruby red grapefruit
1 pint fresh strawberries, rinsed and hulled
1 cup maple sugar
2 tablespoons unsalted butter
4 sprigs fresh mint for garnish

Preheat the broiler.

With a sharp knife, cut the rind and white fleshy membrane from the grapefruit. Carefully separate the grapefruit segments, using a sharp knife and holding the fruit over a small bowl to catch any juice. Squeeze any remaining juice from the trimmed sections.

Combine the strawberries and the grapefruit juice in a blender, puréeing until smooth. Taste for sweetness and add about a tablespoon of the maple sugar if necessary. Strain through a fine sieve to remove the seeds.

Nutritional Analysis per serving

Calories: 346
Good source of vitamin C and moderate source of fiber
Fat: 4.5 g
Saturated fat: 2.4 g
Cholesterol: 10 mg
Sodium: 8 mg

To make the maple sugar crisps, butter a baking sheet. Spoon about 1 tablespoon of the maple sugar onto the baking sheet and spread to the size of a 50-cent piece. Repeat this process with the remaining sugar, leaving room between each one for the sugar to expand when caramelized. Put the baking sheet under the broiler and heat for 2 to 3 minutes, until the sugar is dark brown and caramelized. Rotate the baking sheet as necessary to ensure even caramelization. Remove from the broiler and set the baking sheet on a wire rack to cool. Allow the crisps to cool to room temperature before lifting from the baking sheet with a thin metal spatula.

Arrange the grapefruit segments, alternating between white and ruby, in a circle emanating from the center of each of 4 serving dishes. Spoon the strawberry purée over the grapefruit segments and garnish each plate with a sprig of mint. Top the grapefruit with whole or crumbled sugar crisps. Serve immediately.

LARRY FORGIONE
·····················

FRESH HERB AND SPINACH OMELET
Serves 4

Omelets are traditional favorites for breakfast or brunch—and even for supper. Larry prepares this one with more egg whites than whole eggs to keep the fat and cholesterol counts low.

9 large egg whites
3 large eggs
¼ cup fresh herbs, such as chervil, tarragon, chopped basil, or oregano
4 teaspoons olive oil
1 teaspoon minced garlic
2 cups drained cooked spinach
Kosher salt (optional)
Few grinds fresh black pepper

In a bowl, beat together the egg whites, eggs, and herbs until combined.

In a 6-inch nonstick sauté pan, heat 1 teaspoon of olive oil over medium heat. Add ¼ teaspoon garlic and cook for about 1 minute. Add ½ cup of the spinach and sauté for 1 to 2 minutes. Season to taste with salt and pepper.

Pour a quarter of the egg mixture into the pan on top of the spinach and stir over low heat until the eggs begin to set. At this point, use a spatula to fold over the two sides of the omelet.

Invert the omelet onto a heated plate. Prepare three more omelets using the remaining ingredients in the same amounts.

> *Nutritional Analysis per serving (no salt added)*
>
> *Calories: 164*
> *Fat: 8.5 g*
> *Saturated fat: 1.8 g*
> *Cholesterol: 159 mg*
> *Sodium: 253 mg*
> *Good source of vitamin A and moderate source of fiber.*

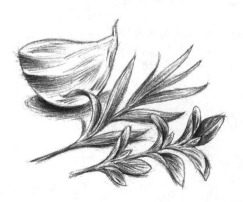

Lunch and Salads

LARRY FORGIONE
....

JICAMA, PINEAPPLE, AND WATERCRESS SALAD
Serves 4

Jicama (pronounced HEE-kah-mah) is a vegetable that is becoming familiar in much of the country, particularly those areas with sizable Latin and Asian populations. Most of the mild-tasting tubers sold in supermarkets and greengrocers' from coast to coast are exported by Mexico, where they are eaten in cooked and raw preparations. They are also commonplace in Chinese cooking and other Eastern cuisines. Look for smooth specimens with thin skin and juicy, ivory-colored flesh. While there really is no substitute, you may use cucumber or apple instead. Larry uses jicama to good advantage in this refreshing, tangy salad nestled on a bed of peppery watercress—one of the first fresh greens of the season. Try this with grilled fish and seafood.

About 2 ounces watercress (2 bunches)
2 cups peeled and thinly sliced jicama (1 jicama), cucumber, or
    tart apple, cut into strips
1 cup thinly sliced red bell pepper (1 pepper), cut into strips
About 8 ounces fresh pineapple (about a quarter of a pineapple)
Juice of 2 limes
2 tablespoons chopped fresh cilantro
1 tablespoon plus 1½ teaspoons extra-virgin olive oil
Kosher salt (optional)
Few grinds fresh black pepper

Wash the watercress and pick the tender branches from the main stems. Arrange these branches in the center of the plate to make a nest. Discard the stems.

Using a sharp knife, peel the pineapple and slice it thin, holding it over a bowl to catch the juices. Cut the slices into strips.

Put the jicama, red bell pepper, and pineapple slices into the bowl holding the pineapple juice and add the lime juice, cilantro, and olive oil. Toss and season to taste with salt and pepper. Let stand for 10 minutes.

Using a slotted spoon, spoon the jicama salad over the watercress and drizzle with the remaining dressing.

Nutritional Analysis per serving (no salt added)

Calories: 110
Fat: 5.5 g
Saturated fat: 0.8 g
Cholesterol: 0 mg
Sodium: 11mg
Source of vitamin C, E, and A and moderate source of fiber

LARRY FORGIONE
....

POACHED OYSTERS AND SHRIMP WITH LEMON-PEPPER DRESSING
Serves 4

This light, cool dish can be made well ahead of time. If you prefer, substitute cooked lobster or crayfish tails for the shrimp. This recipe has a relatively high percentage of calories from fat, but the amount of saturated fat is quite low.

16 oysters, unshucked
2 tablespoons dry white wine
Tabasco
Kosher salt
Few grinds of fresh black pepper
8 ounces fresh small shrimp, cooked and shelled
2 tablespoons chopped parsley

Lemon-Pepper Dressing
2 large egg yolks
½ cup olive oil
3 tablespoons lemon juice
3 tablespoons white wine vinegar
Poaching liquid from oysters
1½ teaspoons fresh black pepper
Grated zest of 2 lemons
¼ teaspoon salt

Shuck the oysters over a small saucepan to catch their liquor. Save the bottom shells.

Add the wine to the oyster liquor and bring to a simmer over medium heat. Add the shucked oysters and a few drops of Tabasco; season to taste with salt and pepper. Poach the oysters for 1 to 2 minutes, just until their edges begin to curl. Pour the oysters and the poaching liquid into a bowl, cover, and refrigerate for at least 1 hour until chilled.

When the oysters are completely chilled, drain the liquid from them to use in the dressing.

To make the dressing, beat the egg yolks until thick and lemon colored. Whisking constantly, add half the oil very slowly. Beat in the lemon juice and vinegar and then the remaining oil. If using right away, stir in the drained liquid from the oysters. Add the pepper and lemon zest and season with salt. If making ahead of time, refrigerate the dressing until ready to serve. Add the drained liquid, pepper, lemon zest, and salt just before serving.

(continued)

Nutritional Analysis per serving (oysters and shrimp only, no salt added)

Calories: 94
Fat: 2.0 g
Saturated fat: 0.6 g
Cholesterol: 140 mg
Sodium: 245 mg
No source of fiber

Nutritional Analysis per serving (2 tablespoons dressing per serving)

Calories: 110
Fair source of vitamin E
Fat: 11.8 g
Saturated fat: 1.8 g
Cholesterol: 123 mg
Sodium: 68 mg
Relatively low source of fiber

Spread shaved ice on serving plates or a platter. Arrange the oyster shells on the ice. Put a poached oyster in each shell and evenly distribute the shrimp among the shells. Spoon about 2 tablespoons of the dressing over each oyster and sprinkle with parsley. Reserve leftover dressing for another use.

LARRY FORGIONE

BAKED HALIBUT FILLETS WITH TOMATOES, CAPERS, AND FRESH HERBS

Serves 4

Cooking fish fillets in the oven is a good way to prepare them without a lot of fat. In this recipe, Larry starts the fish in a hot oven and then turns up the heat further by switching on the broiler while the fish are left in the oven. This recipe would work well with sole, too.

4 (5- to 6-ounce) halibut fillets, skinned and boned
3 tablespoons olive oil
Kosher salt (optional)
Few grinds fresh black pepper
2 tomatoes, peeled, seeded, and diced
2 tablespoons small capers
2 teaspoons minced garlic
2 tablespoons fresh lemon juice
2 tablespoons dry white wine
1 tablespoon chopped fresh oregano
2 tablespoons coarsely chopped Italian flat-leaf parsley

Preheat the oven to 425°F.

Rub the fillets with 1 tablespoon of the olive oil and season generously with salt and pepper. Lay the fillets in a nonstick rectangular baking pan large enough to hold them in a single layer. Place in the center of the oven for 5 to 7 minutes. Leave the fish in the oven and turn the oven temperature to broil. Cook the fish (still in the oven) for about 5 minutes longer, until firm and just beginning to flake.

Meanwhile, mix the tomatoes, capers, garlic, lemon juice, wine, the remaining 2 tablespoons of olive oil, oregano, and parsley in a small saucepan. Bring to a simmer over medium heat and cook for 1 to 2 minutes. Remove from the heat.

Spoon the tomato mixture over the fish and serve immediately.

Nutritional Analysis per serving (no salt added)

Calories: 274
Good source of vitamin E
Fat: 13.7 g
Saturated fat: 1.9 g
Cholesterol: 47 mg
Sodium: 149 mg
Relatively low source of fiber

ALICE WATERS
. . . .
SPRING GREENS AND RADISH SALAD
Serves 4

This simple salad does not make an entire meal but is an excellent accompaniment to grilled fish or poultry or a light pasta dish. Alice takes full advantage of the tender greens springtime has to offer.

1 large shallot, minced (about 1 scant tablespoon)
1 clove garlic, peeled and crushed but intact
2 teaspoons red wine vinegar
1 teaspoon sherry vinegar
Kosher salt (optional)
Few grinds fresh black pepper
¼ cup extra-virgin olive oil
4 large handfuls spring greens, such as chervil, mustard greens, oak leaf
  lettuce, arugula, scallions, and field greens such as miner's lettuce, wild
  mustard flowers, new fennel leaves, fiddlehead ferns, wild radish, wild
  mustard leaves, sorrel, watercress, and frisée
About 30 tiny mild radishes, stems attached
Mustard flowers, for garnish (optional)

Mix the shallot, garlic, and vinegars in a small ceramic or glass bowl. Set aside for 30 minutes.

Discard the garlic and season the vinegar with salt and pepper. Whisking constantly, add the oil to the vinegar until emulsified.

Toss the greens in a salad bowl and dress with the vinaigrette. Scatter radishes over the salad and garnish with mustard flowers, if desired.

Nutritional Analysis per serving (no salt added)

Calories: 146
Fat: 13.8 g
Saturated fat: 1.84 g
Cholesterol: 0 mg
Sodium: 23 mg
Good source of vitamins A, C, and E and moderate source of fiber

ALICE WATERS
. . . .

PASTA WITH BITTER SPRING GREENS
Serves 4

What could be better than spring greens gently wilted with a little garlic and olive oil and then tossed with hot pasta? This truly easy dish can include your own preference for greens and vary with their availability in the market.

1 tablespoon olive oil
1 small yellow onion, peeled and diced
1 clove garlic, peeled and minced
4 large handfuls bitter and sweet greens, such as nettles, pea
   shoots, red and green chard, frisée (curly endive), arugula,
   mizuna, small red mustard, dandelion
½ teaspoon minced fresh thyme
⅛ teaspoon hot red pepper flakes
1¼ teaspoons kosher salt
¼ teaspoon fresh lemon juice
12 ounces dried linguine
1 tablespoon extra-virgin olive oil
4 ounces pecorino or Parmesan cheese
⅔ cup toasted bread crumbs

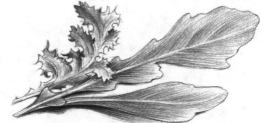

Bring 6 quarts of salted water to a rolling boil in a large pot. Cover and reduce to a simmer.

Heat the olive oil in a large sauté pan. Add the onion, garlic, and 1 tablespoon of water; cover and cook over moderate heat for about 10 minutes, stirring several times, until the onion and garlic are softened. Add the greens, thyme, red pepper flakes, salt, and ½ teaspoon water. Cook, still over moderate heat, turning the greens with tongs, for 2 to 6 minutes, until just wilted. Season with lemon juice and set aside in a warm spot.

Nutritional Analysis per serving

Calories: 531
Fat: 16.3 g
Saturated fat: 6.1 g
Cholesterol: 30 mg
Sodium: 1,179 mg
Good source of vitamins E and A and moderate source of fiber

Bring the 6 quarts of water back to a rolling boil. Drop the pasta in the water and cook for 10 to 12 minutes, until firm and resilient. Drain the pasta and add it to the pan containing the greens. Drizzle with the tablespoon of extra-virgin olive oil and toss together until well mixed.

Transfer to a warm bowl, grate the cheese over the pasta, and scatter the bread crumbs over the top.

JIMMY SCHMIDT
....

RADICCHIO, WATERCRESS, RADISH, AND WALNUT SALAD

Serves 4

Peppery radishes and watercress and bitter radicchio are enhanced by a light vinaigrette and sweet, crunchy toasted walnuts in this salad.

¼ cup (about 2 ounces) shelled walnuts
1 tablespoon fresh lemon juice
¼ cup extra-virgin olive oil
Kosher salt (optional)
Few grinds fresh black pepper
About 4 ounces watercress (4 bunches)
1 small head radicchio
8 radishes, sliced very thin
¼ cup snipped fresh chives

Preheat the oven to 350°F.

Spread the walnuts on a baking sheet and bake for about 15 minutes, until lightly browned and fragrant. Transfer the nuts to another sheet to cool completely.

Whisk together the lemon juice and olive oil in a small bowl. Season to taste with salt and pepper and set the dressing aside.

Trim the stems from the watercress, rinse well, and dry thoroughly. Set aside.

Peel 8 of the large outer leaves from the head of the radicchio. Arrange 2 leaves together to form a cup on each of 4 serving plates.

Cut the remainder of the radicchio, or up to 2 cups, into ¼-inch julienne and put in a medium bowl. Add the watercress, radishes, and dressing and toss well.

Divide the salad among the 4 radicchio cups. Sprinkle with chives and nuts. Season with a little more pepper and serve.

Nutritional Analysis per serving (no added salt)

Calories: 183
Fat: 18.3 g
Saturated fat: 2.3 g
Cholesterol: 0 mg
Sodium: 25 mg
Relatively high in vitamins E and A and relatively low source of fiber

JIMMY SCHMIDT
....

SHRIMP AND SORREL RISOTTO

Serves 4

The rice Jimmy uses here is arborio, the Italian short-grain rice typically used for risotto and sold in nearly every specialty shop and Italian market, as well as many supermarkets across the country. The rice adds to the creamy texture that is so important for authentic risotto. He also relies for flavor on sorrel, a decidedly sour-tasting green used extensively throughout Europe and becoming quite popular here as well. Cultivated sorrel has larger leaves and milder flavor than wild sorrel and is at the peak of its season in late spring and early summer. The chef sometimes makes this with crayfish instead of shrimp, and if you have access to crayfish, try them. The risotto is equally good, and with crayfish, the calorie and fat counts go down a little, too.

¾ cup chopped fresh sorrel plus 4 large sorrel leaves, cut into fine julienne
¼ cup snipped fresh chives
Grated zest of 1 lemon
1 anchovy fillet, mashed with a fork (optional)
4½ cups homemade vegetable broth (see page 194) or low-sodium
    broth from bouillon cubes
2 tablespoons extra-virgin olive oil
1 tablespoon minced garlic
½ cup diced scallions, green and white parts
2 cups arborio rice
2 teaspoons ground turmeric
1½ cups dry white wine
1½ pounds shrimp, shelled and deveined
Kosher salt
Few grinds fresh black pepper

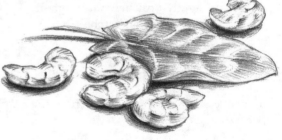

Combine the chopped sorrel, chives, lemon zest, and mashed anchovy in a small bowl and mix well. Set aside.

Gently heat the vegetable broth until it reaches a boil. Keep at a simmer while you prepare the rice.

Heat the olive oil in a deep, heavy saucepan over medium-high heat. Add the garlic and cook for about 2 minutes, until golden. Add the scallions and cook for 1 minute. Stir in the rice and cook for about 2 minutes, until hot. Add the turmeric and white wine and cook for about 4 minutes, stirring occasionally, until the wine is almost completely absorbed.

Nutritional Analysis per serving (risotto with no added salt)

Calories: 558
Fat: 10.6 g
Saturated fat: 1.8 g
Cholesterol: 167 mg
Sodium: 324 mg
Relatively high in vitamins A, E, and C and moderate source of fiber.

Stir in 1 cup of boiling broth and cook for about 4 minutes, stirring
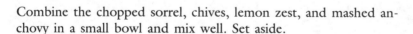
often, until the liquid is almost completely absorbed. Repeat this procedure with all but 1½ cups of the remaining broth. Add the shrimp and the remaining broth and cook for about 3

minutes, until thoroughly heated. Add the chopped sorrel–lemon zest mixture and cook for about 1 minute, until the rice is creamy but no longer loose. Season to taste with salt and pepper.

Spoon the risotto into 4 shallow bowls. Top with the julienned sorrel and serve immediately.

JIMMY SCHMIDT

RAGOUT OF BABY ARTICHOKES AND STUFFED MOREL MUSHROOMS

Serves 4

Roasted garlic and bitter arugula make a filling for tender morels, one of spring's finest offerings. Be sure to pack the filling gently yet securely into the mushroom caps so that it does not fall out during cooking. To complete this full-flavored vegetable dish, Jimmy adds quartered baby artichokes.

1 large whole head garlic, papery outer skin removed
12 baby artichokes
Juice of 2 lemons
½ cup finely chopped arugula
¼ cup chopped flat-leaf parsley
1 tablespoon chopped fresh rosemary
2 tablespoons grated Parmesan cheese
Kosher salt (optional)
Few grinds fresh black pepper
1 pound large morel mushrooms, cleaned and stemmed
Extra-virgin olive oil
1 cup dry sherry
¼ cup snipped fresh chives

Preheat the oven to 400°F.

Put the garlic head in a small, lightly oiled ovenproof dish. Roast the garlic, uncovered, on the lower rack of the oven for about 30 minutes, until the skin is brown and the inside flesh is tender. Remove from the oven and allow to cool to room temperature. Peel to expose the tender inner vegetable or squeeze by hand to force the garlic from the skin. Mash well.

Fill a medium saucepan with water and heat to boiling.

Meanwhile, clean the artichokes by removing the coarse outer leaves and trimming off the stems and the coarse points of the leaves. Squeeze the lemon juice into a large bowl and toss each artichoke in juice as it is trimmed.

Nutritional Analysis per serving

Calories: 201
High in fiber and vitamin C
Fat: 5.3 g
Saturated fat: 1.2 g
Cholesterol: 2 mg
Sodium: 239 mg

(continued)

Cook the artichokes in the boiling water for 10 to 15 minutes, until tender. Drain and set aside at room temperature.

In a small bowl, combine the mashed roasted garlic, arugula, parsley, rosemary, and Parmesan cheese. Season to taste with salt and a generous amount of black pepper.

Invert a morel and spoon the garlic-arugula mixture into the mushroom cap. Pack firmly with the back of a spoon to hold in place. Repeat with the remaining morels.

Heat a large nonstick skillet over medium-high heat. Lightly brush the pan with olive oil. Cook the mushrooms for about 3 minutes until golden. Continue cooking for another 2 minutes, shaking the pan and rolling the morels over to sear them.

Cut the artichokes into quarters lengthwise and add to the mushrooms. Add the sherry and cook for about 3 minutes, until the liquid is reduced and coats the vegetables. Season to taste with salt and pepper. Remove from the heat and add half the chives, tossing to combine.

Place a mound of the artichokes and mushrooms in the center of each of 4 serving plates. Sprinkle with the remaining chives and serve.

Appetizers

LARRY FORGIONE
. . . .

CHILLED OYSTERS WITH A CUCUMBER-MINT SAUCE
Serves 4

Cucumbers combine with fresh mint and cilantro for a fresh-tasting dipping sauce for briny oysters. Shuck the oysters yourself or ask the fishmonger to do it for you. This ensures freshness. Don't buy them already shucked.

½ cup peeled, seeded, and finely diced cucumber
2 tablespoons chopped fresh mint
2 tablespoons chopped fresh cilantro
1 tablespoon coarsely ground black pepper
¼ cup red wine vinegar
24 shucked oysters, chilled

In a bowl, combine the cucumber, mint, cilantro, pepper, and vinegar. Let stand at least 15 to 20 minutes.

Pour the mixture into a serving dish and serve as a dipping sauce with the chilled oysters.

Nutritional Analysis per serving

Calories: 250
Fat: 6.9 g
Saturated fat: 1.5 g
Cholesterol: 149 mg
Sodium: 318 mg
Good source of vitamins E and A, and relatively low source of fiber

JIMMY SCHMIDT
....

GRILLED ASPARAGUS WITH CHERVIL AND HAZELNUTS

Serves 4

Grilling springtime's asparagus is a wonderful way to enjoy it. Asparagus spears snap where they are meant to break if you bend them gently, thus making it unnecessary to cut the tough ends with a knife. In this recipe, Jimmy sprinkles finely chopped toasted hazelnuts over the asparagus. Also called filberts, hazelnuts will be freshest if you buy them in the shell.

¼ cup (about 1 generous ounce) whole hazelnuts
2 pounds asparagus (about 36 jumbo spears)
2 tablespoons extra-virgin olive oil
Kosher salt (optional)
Few grinds fresh black pepper
¼ cup balsamic vinegar
1½ cups fresh chervil sprigs with small stems

Preheat the oven to 350°F.

Spread the hazelnuts on a baking sheet and bake for about 10 minutes, until lightly browned and fragrant. Transfer the nuts to another sheet to cool completely. When cool, rub them between your fingers to remove as much of the skin as possible. Put the nuts in a food processor fitted with the metal blade and process until the size of short-grain rice. Strain the nuts in a large-mesh sieve to remove the small, dustlike particles and set aside.

Prepare a charcoal, wood, or gas grill or preheat the broiler.

Nutritional Analysis per serving (no salt added)

Calories: 115
Moderate source of fiber, and vitamins A, C, and E
Fat: 8.3 g
Saturated fat: 0.9 g
Cholesterol: 0 mg
Sodium: 16 mg

Snap the coarse lower stems from the asparagus and peel the remaining stems if they are tough or gritty.

Place the asparagus in a large bowl and cover with the olive oil, mixing to coat evenly.

Lay the asparagus on the grill. Cook for about 2 minutes, until seared. Using tongs, turn over to finish cooking, about 2 more minutes, until hot but still crunchy. Season to taste with salt and pepper. Alternatively, cook in a preheated broiler 4 to 5 inches from the heat source, turning several times. Do not let them burn.

Divide the spears evenly among 4 plates and arrange them so that the tips point in the same direction. Spoon 1 tablespoon of the balsamic vinegar over the asparagus on each plate. Sprinkle the hazelnuts evenly over the asparagus and season with a little more pepper. Top the asparagus with the chervil and serve.

ALICE WATERS
....

GRILLED YOUNG LEEKS ON TOAST

Serves 4

Alice likes to use fresh fava beans when they come into season in the spring and early summer. Here, she cooks fava beans and mashes them into a purée that, after spreading on toast, she tops with lightly grilled leeks. What a nice way to start a balmy spring evening! Beans are wonderful sources of fiber and supply other necessary nutrients, but don't be fooled into thinking they are low in fat. They have zero cholesterol but a relatively high calorie and fat content.

⅔ cup shelled fresh fava beans
1½ pounds young leeks, about ½ inch in diameter
3 tablespoons extra-virgin olive oil
⅓ teaspoon kosher salt
8 (3- × 2-inch) pieces toasted country-style whole wheat or similar
  bread
8 to 10 anchovy fillets, sliced thin if thick (optional)
Juice of 1 lemon
Few grinds fresh black pepper

In a small saucepan, bring about 3 cups of water to a boil and add the fava beans. Blanch for 2 to 6 minutes, depending on size. Drain and cool. Rub off the skins.

Cut off the root ends of the leeks, leaving as much of the white part as possible. Cut off the green tops just at the point where the stem branches into leaves. Wash thoroughly under cold running water to remove all grit.

Bring about 2 inches of salted water to a boil in a large skillet. Lay the leeks in the pan and poach for 6 to 7 minutes. When ready, the point of a sharp knife should pass easily through the leeks. Lift the leeks from the water with a spatula and lay them in a single layer on a flat plate. Cool in the refrigerator.

Put 1 tablespoon of the olive oil, ¾ cup of water, and the salt in a saucepan and add the skinned fava beans. Cover and cook over moderate heat for about 35 minutes, stirring often, until very soft and the beans can be stirred into a purée with the consistency of lightly whipped cream. Add more water during cooking if necessary.

Take the leeks from the refrigerator and let them come to room temperature. Lightly oil them with about half the remaining oil.

Prepare a charcoal, gas, or wood grill, or preheat the broiler.

Nutritional Analysis per serving (without anchovies)

Calories: 421
Fat: 13.2 g
Saturated fat: 2 g
Cholesterol: 0 mg
Sodium: 464 mg
High in fiber and vitamin E

Nutritional Analysis per serving (with anchovies)

Calories: 437
Fat: 14 g
Saturated fat: 2.2 g
Cholesterol: 7 mg
Sodium: 757 mg
High in fiber and vitamin E

Grill the leeks over moderate heat for 5 to 6 minutes, turning several times, until browned and evenly cooked. Set aside in a warm spot.

Spread the toasts liberally with bean purée and arrange them on a large platter. Split the leeks down the middle and lay them on the toasts. Top with anchovy fillets and drizzle with the remaining oil and the lemon juice. Season with pepper and serve.

Dinner

JIMMY SCHMIDT

HALIBUT, SWEET PEA, AND FINES HERBES STEW

Serves 4

Springtime beckons with just-dug tiny new potatoes, garden-fresh sweet peas, and fresh herbs so superior to those you have used all winter. You will be charmed by Jimmy's simple fish stew bursting with these good things.

2 cups dry white wine
6 cups homemade vegetable broth (page 194) or low-sodium vegetable
    broth made from bouillon cubes or homemade fish or chicken broth
    (pages 195 and 193) or low-sodium canned (chicken) broth
Kosher salt (optional)
Ground red pepper (cayenne)
8 baby new potatoes, skin on, washed (about 8 ounces)
2 cups shelled baby sweet peas
4 (5- to 6-ounce) halibut fillets, trimmed of skin and fat
2 tablespoons snipped fresh chives
3 tablespoons fresh tarragon leaves
1 tablespoon chopped flat-leaf parsley
1 cup chervil sprigs (small stems attached)

Combine the white wine and broth in a nonreactive saucepan and bring to a gentle simmer over medium-high heat. Cook for about 20 minutes, until reduced to about 3 cups. Strain through a very fine sieve, a double thickness of cheesecloth, or a paper coffee filter into a large saucepan or deep skillet. Season to taste with salt and cayenne pepper. Set aside and keep warm.

Meanwhile, steam the potatoes in a steaming basket set over a saucepan of rapidly boiling water. Cook for about 15 minutes, until tender. Lift the potatoes from the basket, let cool slightly, peel, and cut into large dice. Return the diced potatoes to the steamer and add the peas. Cook for about 4 minutes longer, or just until the peas are tender. Remove from the heat.   *(continued)*

Nutritional Analysis per serving (no salt added)

Calories: 409
Good source of fiber and vitamin C
Fat: 6.5 g
Saturated fat: 1.2 g
Cholesterol: 52 mg
Sodium: 238 mg

While the peas cook, set the broth over medium heat. When almost simmering, add the fillets and cook for about 6 minutes (depending on thickness), until opaque and almost flaky. Add the chives, tarragon, and parsley, stirring to combine. Add the potatoes and peas and remove the pan from the heat.

Set the halibut on a serving platter or on 4 individual plates. Spoon the potatoes and peas around the fish. Spoon the broth over the halibut and top with chervil. Serve immediately.

JIMMY SCHMIDT

CHICKEN GRILLED WITH CITRUS, ROASTED GARLIC, AND ARTICHOKES
Serves 4

Lemons, roasted garlic, and thyme combine in this tantalizing dish of tender spring chickens grilled to a moist turn and served with baby artichokes. You might want to ask the butcher to bone the chickens for you by first splitting them down the back. Small, one-pound chickens are sometimes called *poussin*. You can substitute Cornish game hens for chicken in this recipe.

3 large whole heads of garlic, outside papery husks removed
Olive oil
4 lemons
Few grinds fresh pepper
4 (1-pound) chickens, boned except for wing tips and drumsticks
2 tablespoons virgin olive oil
12 medium baby artichokes
1 cup dry vermouth
2 cups homemade vegetable broth (see page 194) or low-sodium
  vegetable broth made from bouillon cubes
1 tablespoon chopped fresh thyme leaves
Sea salt (optional)
4 sprigs fresh thyme or other herb for garnish

Preheat the oven to 400°F.

In an ovenproof dish, rub the garlic with just enough oil to coat it. Set the dish on the lower rack of the oven and cook about 30 minutes, until the skin is brown and the inside flesh is tender. Remove from the oven and allow to cool to room temperature. Peel one head only to expose the tender inner vegetable or squeeze by hand to force the garlic from the skin. Mash well. You will have about ¼ cup mashed garlic. Reserve the other 2 heads intact.

Prepare a charcoal, wood, or gas grill or preheat the broiler.

Peel the zest from the lemons and chop it well. Squeeze the juice from the lemons and set aside.

In a small bowl, mix the chopped zest with the ¼ cup mashed roasted garlic and a generous amount of black pepper. Rub this mixture under the skin of the chickens. Rub the outside of the chickens with olive oil and season with black pepper. Put the chickens in a shallow pan and refrigerate for at least 1 hour.

Clean the artichokes by removing the coarse outer leaves and trimming off the stems and the coarse points of the leaves. Cut each one in half lengthwise and immediately toss with the lemon juice to cover all surfaces. Repeat with the remaining artichokes.

Combine the artichokes, lemon juice, and vermouth in a medium nonreactive saucepan and bring to a simmer over medium-high heat. Cover and cook for about 5 minutes, until the liquid is almost completely reduced. Add the broth and cook the artichokes for about 8 minutes, or until tender. Add the remaining 2 heads of roasted garlic, divided into cloves, raise the heat, and cook for about 3 minutes, until the liquid thickens enough to coat the back of a spoon.

Add the thyme and season as necessary with salt and pepper. Keep warm while the chicken is cooking.

Grill or broil the chicken, skin side facing the heat, for about 5 minutes, until seared and golden. Turn over and cook another 6 minutes, depending on the size of the chicken, until done. Spoon some of the artichokes into the center of each of 4 serving plates, reserving about a quarter of the mixture. Remove the skin from the chicken, if you prefer, at this point. Place the chicken over the artichokes and spoon the remaining sauce over it. Garnish with the sprigs of thyme and serve.

Nutritional Analysis per serving (5 ounces of skinless chicken, no salt added)

Calories: 501
High source of fiber and good source of vitamin C
Fat: 11.4 g
Saturated fat: 3.1 g
Cholesterol: 128 mg
Sodium: 171 mg

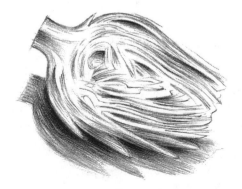

JIMMY SCHMIDT
....

RACK OF LAMB WITH JERUSALEM ARTICHOKES AND MINT
Serves 4

Rack of lamb is an elegant way to serve lamb. Once cooked, it is cut into small but exquisitely tasty rib lamb chops. In this recipe, Jimmy makes a ragout from Jerusalem artichokes and potatoes and a sauce from mint leaves. Both the ragout and the mint sauce are flavored with soft, cooked garlic.

1 (6- to 7-pound) rack of lamb with 8 bones, trimmed (see Note)
Salt (optional) and freshly ground black pepper
1 large head of garlic, cut in half horizontally (on the equator)
8 Jerusalem artichokes (about 1 pound)
8 small new potatoes (about 8 ounces)
1 cup dry white wine, such as Chardonnay
½ cup vegetable broth (page 194)
1 cup stemmed fresh mint leaves
4 sprigs fresh mint for garnish

Preheat the oven to 400°F.

Season the lamb with salt and pepper and put it in a roasting pan with the head of garlic. Roast on the lowest rack of the oven for 35 to 45 minutes, or until a meat thermometer inserted in the meat, without touching the bone, reads 130°F for medium-rare meat. Remove from the oven, transfer the garlic to a plate, cover the lamb loosely with foil, and set aside at room temperature. Do not turn off the oven.

When the garlic is cool enough to handle, squeeze the pulp from the skins and discard the skins. Set the garlic pulp aside.

Nutritional Analysis per serving (fat trimmed, no salt added)

Calories: 585
Fat: 22.8 g
Saturated fat: 8.1 g
Cholesterol: 150 mg
Sodium: 216 mg
Moderate source of fiber.

In a large saucepan, cook the Jerusalem artichokes and potatoes in lightly salted boiling water for 30 to 40 minutes, or until fork tender. Drain and cool. When cool enough to handle, peel the artichokes and cut them into thin slices. Peel the potatoes and cut them into cubes.

Transfer a quarter of the artichokes and half the garlic to a blender or food processor and purée, adding up to ½ cup of the wine, until smooth.

Transfer the purée to a nonstick skillet and add the broth and the remaining Jerusalem artichokes. Bring to a simmer over medium-high heat and cook for about 5 minutes, or until thickened to sauce consistency. Add the potatoes and heat until warmed. Season to taste with salt and pepper. Remove from the heat and cover to keep warm.

In a blender, combine the mint leaves, the remaining garlic, and the remaining wine. Purée until smooth. Season to taste with salt and pepper.

Return the lamb to the oven and reheat for about 5 minutes until hot. Using a sharp knife, cut the lamb between the bones to separate into chops. Spoon the Jerusalem artichoke and potato ragout onto each plate and arrange the chops next to it. Drizzle the lamb and the ragout with mint sauce and garnish each plate with a mint sprig.

Note: Ask the butcher to trim the rack of lamb by removing the fat covering the meat and between the bones. Or do it yourself using a small sharp knife.

ALICE WATERS

BAKED SALMON WITH WATERCRESS SAUCE
Serves 4

Salmon and watercress are rites of spring as certainly as are tulips and gentle rain. Alice makes a simple watercress sauce that accentuates the goodness of the salmon. The result is an elegant dish that is very low in saturated fat and calories.

4 (5-ounce) salmon fillets, about 1 inch thick
Kosher salt (optional) and freshly ground pepper
2 bunches watercress
1 tablespoon extra-virgin olive oil
Juice of about ½ lemon or about 1 tablespoon white wine vinegar

Preheat the oven to 400°F.

Sprinkle each fillet on both sides with a little salt and pepper. Set aside and allow the salmon to reach room temperature.

Pick over and rinse the watercress, selecting only the leaves and small, tender stems. Put the watercress in a strainer.

Nutritional Analysis per serving (no salt added)

Calories: 289
Fat: 16.9 g
Saturated fat: 2.8 g
Cholesterol: 99 mg
Sodium: 85 mg
Good source of vitamin E and A and relatively low source of fiber

Select a saucepan large enough to hold the strainer and fill it about two-thirds full with water. Bring to a rolling boil. Have ready a 3-quart bowl full of ice and water. When the water in the saucepan is boiling, submerge the watercress and strainer into it for about 30 seconds. Lift the strainer from the water and immediately plunge it in the ice water bath to cool, stop the cooking, and preserve the color of the cress. Lift the strainer from the water bath and let the watercress drain.

Put the watercress and a teaspoon of olive oil in a blender or food processor and purée until smooth. Add the lemon juice, a few drops at a time, and a pinch of salt to taste. Keep the sauce at room temperature.

Lightly oil a baking sheet with the remaining olive oil and lay the salmon fillets on it. Bake the fish for about 12 minutes, until just pink in the center. Transfer to a warm platter and top each fillet with a little of the watercress sauce.

ALICE WATERS
·····················

SPRING TURNIP SOUP
Serves 4

This puréed soup makes a delightful supper served with a green salad and a loaf of bread. It would also make a nice first course or lunch dish. Alice likes to use young turnips, which are about 2 to 3 inches in diameter. The little turnips are attached to leaves that are about eight inches long. Buy them with the leaves, as the leaves are used in the soup, too. If you cannot find baby turnips, use the freshest-looking turnips you can find. This recipe is exceptionally low in total and saturated fat.

1½ teaspoons olive oil
1 yellow onion, peeled and sliced thin
1 small rib celery, diced
¾ pound young turnips with greens (about 1 large bunch)
¼ teaspoon finely chopped fresh thyme leaves
4 cups homemade chicken broth (page 193) or low-sodium canned broth
Kosher salt
Few grinds fresh black pepper
½ teaspoon red wine vinegar

Heat half the olive oil and 1 tablespoon water in a large, deep saucepan. Add the onion and celery and cook over medium heat for about 10 minutes, until the vegetables are soft and translucent.

Remove the leaves from the turnips and set aside. Chop the turnips coarse and add them to the pan with the thyme, chicken broth, and salt and pepper to taste. Bring to a boil, then reduce the heat to a simmer. Cover and cook over low heat for 1 hour.

Nutritional Analysis per serving (no salt added)

Calories: 74
Fat: 3.2 g
Saturated fat: 0.6 g
Cholesterol: 0 mg
Sodium: 103 mg
Relatively low source of fiber

Purée the soup in a blender or food processor until smooth. If using a blender, you may have to purée it in batches. Strain through a fine mesh strainer into the saucepan. Adjust the seasonings and add the vinegar.

Chop the reserved turnip leaves fine. Heat 3 tablespoons of water and a little salt in a small saucepan and cook the chopped leaves for about 5 minutes over medium heat.

Bring the soup to a simmer. Stir in the greens and serve immediately.

LARRY FORGIONE
....

GRILLED CHICKEN, FOREST MUSHROOMS, AND RED ONION PASTA

Serves 4

In this recipe, which combines the sweetness of red onions with the earthiness of shiitake mushrooms, chicken is first grilled and then sautéed before being served over hot pasta. Substitute another type of mushroom if you prefer. While the fat content is relatively high, the saturated fat content is not.

12 ounces dried penne
2 (8-ounce) boned and skinned chicken breast halves
12 shiitake or other wild mushrooms
1 red onion, peeled and cut into ½-inch slices
3 tablespoons extra-virgin olive oil
Kosher salt (optional)
Few grinds fresh black pepper
2 teaspoons minced garlic
1 large ripe tomato, peeled, seeded, and chopped
16 snow peas, cut at an angle into lengthwise strips
1½ teaspoons chopped fresh marjoram
1 tablespoon chopped parsley
1 cup homemade chicken broth (page 193) or low-sodium canned broth

Prepare a charcoal, wood, or gas grill or preheat the broiler.

Bring a large saucepan of water to a boil. Cook the penne for 10 to 12 minutes, until firm and resilient. Drain and set aside.

Brush the chicken breasts, mushrooms, and onion slices with some of the olive oil and season to taste with salt and pepper.

Grill the chicken breasts over medium-hot coals for about 3 minutes on each side for medium-rare to medium meat. Grill the mushrooms for 1 minute to a side and the onion slices for 3 minutes to a side. Set all the vegetables aside to cool to room temperature.

Nutritional Analysis per serving (without added salt)

Calories: 606
Fat: 15.2 g
Saturated fat: 2.6 g
Cholesterol: 72 mg
Sodium: 270 mg
Good source of fiber

Using a sharp knife, cut the chicken breasts and mushrooms into thin strips. Cut each onion ring in half.

Heat the remaining olive oil in a large skillet. Add the garlic, chicken, mushrooms, onions, chopped tomato, snow peas, and herbs. Sauté over medium-high heat for about 1 minute. Add the pasta and chicken broth. Bring to a boil and ladle into shallow soup bowls.

LARRY FORGIONE
. . . .

PASTA WITH GRILLED SALMON AND GARLIC BROCCOLI

Serves 4

Larry serves flaked grilled salmon with a pasta toss of broccoli, garlic, and herbs for a pleasing one-dish meal that tastes good and fresh on a spring night. If you leave off the croutons, you save significantly on calories and fat.

4 (4-ounce) skinless, boneless salmon fillets
Kosher salt (optional)
Few grinds fresh black pepper
2 tablespoons olive oil
1 red onion, peeled and cut crosswise into slices
Pinch hot red pepper flakes
3 cups fresh broccoli florets, cooked until crisp-tender
1 tablespoon minced garlic
¾ pound orecchiette pasta, cooked until firm and resilient
2 tablespoons chopped fresh oregano
2 tablespoons chopped parsley
1¼ cups homemade fish or chicken broth (pages 195 and 193) or low-sodium
    canned chicken broth
2 cups fresh croutons (optional)

Prepare a charcoal, wood, or gas grill or preheat the broiler.

Season the salmon with salt and pepper. Rub each fillet with a little olive oil, using about 1 tablespoon of oil. Grill the salmon for 2 minutes on each side. Remove from the heat and cool to room temperature. When the fish is cool enough to handle, flake into large pieces.

Put the remaining olive oil in a large skillet or wok and heat until very hot. Carefully add the red onion and red pepper flakes and stir for 1 minute. Add the broccoli and garlic and stir for 1 minute more. Add the pasta, oregano, parsley, and broth and season with salt and freshly ground black pepper. Stir gently until heated and well combined.

Add the flaked salmon, together with any juice from the fish. Toss gently and spoon into shallow soup bowls.

Sprinkle with croutons before serving, if desired.

Nutritional Analysis per serving (without salt or croutons)

Calories: 604
High in vitamins C, A, and E and a good source of fiber
Fat: 18.2 g
Saturated fat: 2.9 g
Cholesterol: 74 mg
Sodium: 118 mg

LARRY FORGIONE

GAME HENS WITH COUNTRY HAM AND GREENS STUFFING AND BOURBON GLAZE

Serves 4

Boned game hens stuffed with wilted greens make a country-style meal with cosmopolitan flair. The greens are particularly tender in the springtime and lend flavor to the meat. Ask the butcher to bone the hens for you if you are not sure you can do it yourself.

6 ounces young mustard greens or Swiss chard
12 ounces young spinach
1 tablespoon plus 1½ teaspoons peanut oil
1 teaspoon minced garlic
⅓ cup minced onion
¾ cup finely diced country ham
Kosher salt
Few grinds fresh black pepper
Cornish game hens, boned (drumsticks and wing tips left in)

Bourbon Glaze
2 tablespoons bourbon whiskey
2 tablespoons prepared mustard
⅓ cup honey

Preheat the oven to 450°F.

Wash and thoroughly dry the greens and kale and tear into manageable pieces.

Heat the oil in a large skillet over medium heat and add the garlic and onion. Cook for 1 to 2 minutes, stirring. Add the greens and kale and cook for 2 to 3 minutes longer until the greens wilt. Add the ham and season to taste with salt and pepper. Cook for another minute and set aside to cool to room temperature.

Lay the birds on a work surface, skin side down. Fill the thighs with stuffing mixture. Divide the rest of the stuffing into 4 oval portions and mound onto the centers of the birds. Bring the skin up over the stuffing, overlapping it on one side. With a trussing needle, sew up the birds, starting at the necks. Use your hands to shape the birds as much as possible into their original shape. Truss the legs closed so that they resemble whole birds. Season to taste with salt and pepper. Arrange the hens in a roasting pan and cook for 2 to 3 minutes. While the birds roast, combine the glaze ingredients. Brush the glaze over the birds and cook for 5 minutes longer.

(continued)

Nutritional Analysis per serving (with skin and glaze consumed, no salt added)

Calories: 981
Fat: 49 g
Saturated fat: 12.9 g
Cholesterol: 282 mg
Sodium: 1,452 mg
Source of vitamins E, C, and A and fiber

Nutritional Analysis per serving (without skin, no salt added)

Calories: 724
High in vitamins A, E, and C and fiber
Fat: 25.9 g
Saturated fat: 6.49 g
Cholesterol: 234 mg
Sodium: 1,283 mg

Take the birds from the oven. Turn on the broiler. Brush the birds with more glaze and broil for about 1 minute, until glossy. Let the hens rest for 3 to 4 minutes and remove strings and trussing. Serve hot or at room temperature.

Dessert

LARRY FORGIONE
....

CHOCOLATE CHERRY FUDGE CAKE

Makes 10-inch cake; serves 12

This chocolate cake is not a miracle confection without calories or fat. This is a bonafide rich, moist chocolate cake made with a whole pound of chocolate! We included it for several reasons. First, it is delicious. Second, we want to demonstrate that you can have your cake and fat budget, too. If you eat a slice of this cake, limit your intake of fat for the next day or two to compensate for the indulgence. It's worth it!

13 ounces semisweet chocolate, coarsely chopped
3 ounces unsweetened chocolate, coarsely chopped
8 ounces (2 sticks) unsalted butter
1 cup unsweetened cocoa powder
7 large eggs
1½ cups sugar
1 cup dried tart cherries
Confectioners' sugar

Preheat the oven to 350°F. Lightly butter and flour a 10-inch springform pan. Wrap the bottom and outer side of the pan with aluminum foil to prevent leakage. Or lightly butter and flour a 10-inch round cake pan.

Combine the chocolate and the butter in the top of a double boiler and stir over simmering, not boiling, water until almost melted. Remove from the heat and stir until completely melted. Stir in the cocoa.

Combine the eggs and sugar in another bowl and beat with a hand-held electric mixer or whisk over hot water for 2 to 3 minutes, until the mixture is warm. The bottom of the bowl may touch the water. Remove from the heat and continue to beat for 3 to 4 minutes with an electric mixer until the batter triples in volume. Fold in the chocolate mixture and then the dried cherries.

Pour the batter into the prepared pan and set the cake pan in a roasting pan. Pour enough boiling water into the roasting pan to come halfway up the side of the cake pan. Be sure the water does not come over the top of the foil if you are using a springform pan. Bake for 30 to 35 minutes or until a toothpick inserted in the center of the cake comes out clean.

Nutritional Analysis per serving

Calories: 517
Fat: 33.3 g
Saturated fat: 19.3 g
Cholesterol: 168 mg
Sodium: 46 mg
High in fiber and a good source of vitamin A

Allow the cake to cool completely. Release the sides of the springform pan and unmold the cake, or invert the cake pan onto a plate and unmold the cake. Dust with confectioners' sugar before serving.

ALICE WATERS
....

STRAWBERRY GRANITA

Serves 4

When strawberries are ripe and ready for picking, make this icy granita with sweet, juicy berries. It's important to stir the granita as it freezes, as instructed in the recipe. Otherwise, the dessert will freeze into a hard, watery block. The stirring incorporates air so that the granita is the consistency of sorbet. The sugar adds what additional calories there are in this fat-free dessert.

About 4 cups ripe strawberries (two 1-pint baskets)
About ⅓ cup superfine sugar

Trim the strawberries, discarding the hulls and any blemished areas of fruit. Purée the berries in a blender or food processor until smooth.

Strain the purée into a bowl through cheesecloth or a fine sieve, pushing it with the back of a spoon to remove the tiny seeds and thick pulp. Set the purée aside.

Combine ⅓ cup of water with the sugar in a small saucepan and cook over medium heat for about 5 minutes, until the mixture thickens to a light syrupy consistency. Add enough syrup to the strawberry purée to make it the consistency of half-and-half. Taste for sweetness and add more sugar if necessary. Do not add too much sugar, or the granita will not freeze properly.

Nutritional Analysis per serving (granita only)

Calories: 109
Good source of vitamin C and relatively low in fiber
Fat: 0.5 g
Saturated fat: 0.3 g
Cholesterol: 0 mg
Sodium: 2 mg

Scrape the sweetened purée into a 9- or 10-inch square metal pan that is 3 inches deep. Put the pan in the freezer for 30 minutes until the purée begins to freeze. Remove the pan from the freezer, break up the purée with a fork, and stir until smooth. Return the pan to the freezer. Repeat the process every 20 minutes for 2 hours, until the granita is completely frozen and the ice crystals are smaller than crushed ice.

Serve the granita immediately with blood oranges or other spring fruit, or store it, covered, in the freezer for up to 4 hours.

JIMMY SCHMIDT

LOW-FAT CHOCOLATE BROWNIES

Makes about 20 small brownies

These brownies have no butter but still have a pure, rich chocolate flavor. The applesauce adds moistness and extra sweetness. For variety, bake them in a 10-inch round cake pan and cut them into wedges for serving—especially tasty with fresh fruit. We make no claims that these are a super-low-fat treat, but for a satisfying chocolate hit, they work well without too much damage. Just adjust your fat intake for the next day or two. If you choose to include the optional bittersweet chocolate, the calorie count per brownie climbs to 213 and the fat content to 8.6 g, with 3.5 g of saturated fat.

2 ounces unsweetened chocolate, coarsely chopped
2 teaspoons pure vanilla extract
1½ cups granulated sugar
¼ teaspoon salt
3 large eggs, lightly beaten
2 large egg whites, lightly beaten
¾ cup pure maple syrup or honey
1 cup unsweetened applesauce
¼ cup canola oil
1 cup sifted cake flour
¾ cup unsweetened cocoa powder
6 ounces bittersweet chocolate, coarsely chopped (optional)
Confectioners' sugar

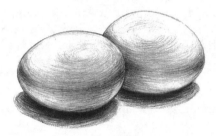

Preheat the oven to 350°F. Lightly coat a 9-inch-square baking pan with vegetable oil spray and line the bottom with parchment paper.

Melt the unsweetened chocolate with the vanilla in the top part of a double boiler set over barely simmering water. Transfer the melted chocolate and vanilla to a large mixing bowl and let cool slightly. Mix in the sugar, salt, eggs, and egg whites, stirring until smooth. Add the syrup, applesauce, and oil and blend until smooth.

Sift the flour and cocoa over the batter and carefully fold in until smooth. Add the chopped chocolate, if desired, and gently fold just to combine. Do not overmix.

Nutritional Analysis per serving (without bittersweet chocolate)

Calories: 173
Fat: 5.5 g
Saturated fat: 1.6 g
Cholesterol: 28 mg
Sodium: 43 mg
Relatively low source of fiber

Pour and scrape the batter into the prepared pan and bake for about 45 minutes, until a toothpick or skewer inserted near the center comes out clean. Set the pan on a wire rack to cool. Dust with confectioners' sugar and cut into squares before serving.

SUMMER RECIPES

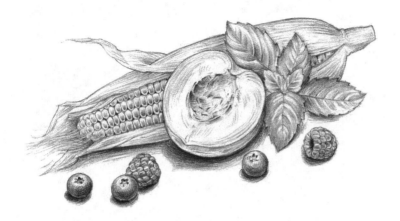

Breakfast

ALICE WATERS
....

MILLET MUFFINS WITH FRESH CORN

Serves 4

Summertime is the only time good fresh corn is available, and Alice uses it in as many ways as possible. For these muffins, she suggests using Silver Queen sweet corn or another variety with small kernels. She also uses millet, a tiny grass seed that adds a slightly toasty flavor and gentle crunch and is also a good source of protein. This recipe makes twelve muffins, which means you will probably have leftover muffins. Wrap them well in plastic and foil and freeze the muffins for up to a month. Thaw them at room temperature.

Scant ¾ cup packed light brown sugar
1 large egg
⅓ cup safflower or corn oil
1 cup buttermilk
7 tablespoons millet (available in natural food stores)
1⅓ cups unbleached all-purpose flour
1 teaspoon baking powder
1 teaspoon baking soda
¼ teaspoon salt
1 cup plus 1 tablespoon fresh corn kernels

Preheat the oven to 375°F. Lightly oil or spray a 12-cup muffin tin with nonstick vegetable oil spray.

Beat the sugar and egg together until smooth. Add the oil and ½ cup of the buttermilk and stir until well blended.

Using a food processor, blender, or mortar and pestle, grind the millet until it is the coarseness of kosher salt.

Whisk the flour with the baking powder, baking soda, and salt. Add the millet and whisk several times to blend.

*Nutritional Analysis
per muffin*

*Calories: 199
Good source of vita-
min E
Fat: 9.3 g
Saturated Fat: 1.1 g
Cholesterol: 18 mg
Sodium: 180 mg
Relatively low source
of fiber*

Add the dry ingredients to the wet ingredients and combine with a few swift strokes. Add the remaining ½ cup of buttermilk and the corn kernels and mix well with a rubber spatula.

Spoon the batter into the muffin cups, filling each one about two-thirds full. Bake for about 22 minutes, until lightly browned and risen. The tops may crack, which is acceptable, and a toothpick inserted in the center of a muffin should come out clean. Cool slightly and then turn out of the muffin tin onto wire racks to cool completely. Serve at room temperature.

JIMMY SCHMIDT
....

SUMMER BERRY AND MAPLE PANCAKES

Serves 4

Just-picked blueberries and raspberries in all their colorful splendor are in now in the markets, and what better way to take advantage of the too-short season than to eat them for breakfast, lunch, and dinner? Here, Jimmy infuses pure maple syrup with blueberries to make a delicious topping for pancakes, which he then serves with fresh raspberries and more blueberries. The topping can be made ahead of time and refrigerated.

¾ cup unbleached all-purpose flour
½ cup whole wheat flour
1 tablespoon baking powder
Pinch kosher salt
1 teaspoon ground cinnamon
1 large egg, beaten
1 to 1¼ cups low-fat milk
3 tablespoons low-fat sour cream
1 cup pure maple syrup
1 pint blueberries
1 cup raspberries
Canola oil
Confectioners' sugar
4 sprigs fresh mint

Whisk together the flours, baking powder, salt, and cinnamon in a large bowl. In another bowl, mix together the egg, milk, and sour cream. Slowly pour the liquid ingredients into the dry ingredients, stirring until just combined. Set aside at room temperature.

Combine the syrup and ½ cup of water in a medium saucepan. Bring to a simmer over medium heat. Add ½ cup of the blueberries to the syrup and cook for about 2 minutes, until just softened. Set a colander over a large bowl. Lift the berries from the saucepan with a slotted spoon and transfer them to the colander to drain. Cook the syrup for about 3 minutes until it is reduced to its original consistency. Add another ½ cup of blueberries and repeat the process. Continue to do this until all the blueberries are cooked and draining in the colander.

Pour the collected blueberry juice from the bowl into the saucepan and bring the syrup to a boil. Cook for about 5 minutes, until thick enough to coat the back of a spoon.

Remove from the heat. Add the cooked blueberries and half of the raspberries. Keep warm or refrigerate if you plan to serve later. If so, bring the syrup to room temperature before serving.

*Nutritional Analysis
per serving*

Calories: 514
Good source of fiber
Fat: 8.9 g
Saturated Fat: 2.1 g
Cholesterol: 54 mg
Sodium: 420 mg

Heat a large, heavy nonstick skillet over medium heat. Carefully brush the skillet with just enough canola oil to coat it lightly. Spoon about ¼ cup of the batter into the skillet to form a 4-inch pancake. Bake for about 2 minutes, until the surface begins to bubble and the bottom is browned.

Turn over and bake for about 1 minute, until cooked through. Remove to a plate and keep warm in the oven while using the rest of the pancake batter.

Divide the pancakes among 4 serving plates. Spoon the room-temperature berry compote across the pancakes. Sprinkle with the remaining raspberries. Top with a shake of confectioners' sugar and garnish with a sprig of mint.

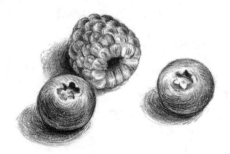

LARRY FORGIONE
....

SUMMER VEGETABLE FRITTATA
Serves 4

This frittata takes full advantage of the summer garden's crops, from new potatoes and tomatoes to summer sweet corn. Larry supplies a recipe for fresh salsa, although you could use your favorite store-bought salsa if you prefer. The chef's salsa will keep in the refrigerator for up to eight hours. Store in a tightly lidded container.

Salsa
2 ripe tomatoes, peeled, seeded, and diced fine (about 1 cup)
3 tablespoons finely diced red onion
½ small red bell pepper, cored, seeded and diced fine (about ¼ cup)
½ green poblano pepper, cored, seeded, and diced fine (about ¼ cup)
½ jalapeño pepper, cored, seeded, and diced fine
¼ cucumber, peeled, seeded, and diced fine (about ½ cup)
2 tablespoons fresh lime juice
3 tablespoons chopped fresh cilantro
2 to 3 drops Tabasco
Pinch sugar
Few grinds fresh black pepper

Frittata
8 small new potatoes
1 cup yellow wax beans, topped and tailed
½ cup shelled fresh peas or frozen peas
1 tablespoon olive oil
2 small onions, sliced
1 small zucchini, diced
1 small yellow squash, diced
1 cup diced yellow plum tomato (2 to 3 plum tomatoes)
1 cup fresh corn kernels, cut from the cob (2 to 3 ears)
Kosher salt (optional)
Few grinds fresh black pepper
3 large eggs, beaten
2 tablespoons chopped fresh herbs, such as chervil, tarragon, basil, or oregano
1 cup grated low-fat mozzarella or jack cheese

To make the salsa, combine the tomatoes, onion, diced peppers, and cucumber in a bowl. Add the lime juice and cilantro and season to taste with Tabasco, sugar, and ground pepper. Mix well. Let the salsa stand in a cool place for at least 30 minutes before serving. This makes about 1 cup of salsa.

To make the frittata, bring a large pot of water to a boil and cook the potatoes for about 20 minutes, until fork tender. Drain and set aside to cool.

Preheat the oven to 350°F.

Bring a smaller saucepan of water to a boil and cook the wax beans for 2 to 3 minutes, just until crisp-tender. Drain and set aside. Cook the peas in boiling water to cover for 2 to 3 minutes, taking care not to overcook; they should be firm. Drain and set aside.

When the potatoes are cool enough, peel them and cut into quarters. Cut the wax beans into 1-inch lengths.

Heat the olive oil in a 10-inch nonstick ovenproof skillet over high heat. Add the onion, zucchini, yellow squash, tomatoes, corn, potatoes, beans, and peas. Season to taste with salt and pepper. Cook, stirring, for 1 to 2 minutes until the onions just begin to soften.

Pour the beaten eggs and herbs over the vegetables. Lower the heat to medium and, using a wooden spoon or spatula, stir the eggs until they begin to set slightly. Add the cheese and stir to mix well. Smooth the mixture with the back of the spoon.

Put the skillet in the oven and bake for 12 to 15 minutes, until the frittata is set and lightly browned around the edges. Remove from the oven and carefully invert onto a serving platter. Cut the frittata into quarters and serve with the salsa.

Nutritional Analysis per serving (without added salt)

Calories: 357
Fat: 12.9 g
Saturated Fat: 4.7 g
Cholesterol: 175 mg
Sodium: 372 mg
Excellent source of vitamins A and C and fiber

Lunch and Salads

JIMMY SCHMIDT
....

SLICED TOMATOES, GRILLED ONION, AND FRIED BASIL
Serves 4

Jimmy takes full advantage of the season's tomatoes and basil with this simple recipe for onion and tomato salad. The fried basil leaves and the basil-enriched oil heighten the flavor of the salad as plain basil would not. If you have extra basil oil, refrigerate it in a clean, tightly lidded glass jar for up to two weeks. And of course, reducing the amount you use reduces the calorie and total fat count. The onions may take a little more or less time on the grill, depending on their thickness.

1 cup extra-virgin olive oil
1 cup whole fresh basil leaves
2 cloves garlic, peeled and sliced thin
2 Vidalia or other sweet onions, peeled and cut into 8 (½-inch) slices
3 large ripe tomatoes, cut into 12 (½-inch) slices
Kosher salt (optional)
¼ cup sherry vinegar or red wine vinegar
Few coarse grinds fresh black pepper

Heat the olive oil in a small saucepan over medium-high heat. Add ¾ cup of the basil leaves and cook for about 1 minute, until crisp. Using a slotted spoon, transfer to a paper towel–lined plate to drain. Set aside at room temperature.

Remove the saucepan from the heat and immediately add the garlic slices, letting them cook in the hot oil for about 2 minutes, until tender. Using a slotted spoon, transfer the garlic to a paper towel–lined plate to drain. Set aside.

Let the oil cool to room temperature. Transfer to a blender and add the remaining ¼ cup of basil leaves. Purée until smooth and set aside.

Nutritional Analysis per serving (no salt added)

Calories: 228
Fat: 20.7 g
Saturated Fat: 2.8 g
Cholesterol: 0 mg
Sodium: 11 mg
Moderate source of vitamins C and E and fiber

Prepare a charcoal, wood, or gas grill or preheat the broiler. Rub the onion slices with the basil-flavored oil. Place the onions on the grill and sear for about 4 minutes, until well marked. Turn over and cook for about 3 minutes longer, until tender. Remove from the grill and allow to cool to room temperature.

Arrange 2 slices of onion alternating with 3 slices of tomato on each plate, slipping a few slices of garlic between the vegetables. Season the tomatoes with a pinch of salt. Spoon 1 tablespoon each of the vinegar and the basil-flavored oil over the tomatoes and the onions. Season to taste with pepper and top the vegetables with the fried basil. Serve immediately.

JIMMY SCHMIDT

SEA SCALLOPS, RED PEPPERS, AND MARJORAM ANGEL HAIR PASTA

Serves 4

This combination of roasted red peppers and pasta tossed with scallops is perfect on a summer's day. Do not overcook the pasta—in this dish, it finishes cooking with the sauce.

4 red bell peppers
Kosher salt (optional)
2 tablespoons extra-virgin olive oil
1 tablespoon minced garlic
¼ teaspoon hot red pepper flakes or hot Hungarian paprika
3 tablespoons fresh marjoram leaves
1 cup dry white wine, preferably Sauvignon Blanc
1 cup bottled clam juice
1 pound large sea scallops, rinsed, trimmed of small muscle attached to
    side, and patted dry; sliced horizontally, if large
8 ounces dried angel hair pasta
Few grinds fresh black pepper
2 tablespoons snipped fresh chives

Roast the peppers by placing them whole on an open gas flame, an outdoor grill, or under the broiler. Cook, rotating on all sides, for about 10 minutes until the skins are black. Put the peppers in a bowl and cover with plastic wrap. Allow to cool for 15 minutes. Using your hands, peel off the charred skin. Discard the cores, stems, and seeds. Dice the roasted peppers and set aside.

Bring a large pot of salted water to a boil over high heat.

Meanwhile, heat the olive oil in a medium skillet over medium-high heat. Add the garlic and cook for about 2 minutes, until golden. Add the pepper flakes and marjoram and cook for 1 minute, until softened. Add the diced roasted peppers, white wine, and clam juice and cook for about 5 minutes, until the liquid is reduced by half. Take the pan from the heat but keep warm.

Nutritional Analysis per serving (no salt added)

Calories: 417
Excellent source of vitamins A and C
Fat: 12.4 g
Saturated Fat: 1.8 g
Cholesterol: 29 mg
Sodium: 295 mg
Moderate source of fiber and vitamin E

Heat a medium nonstick skillet over medium-high heat. Brush the pan with just enough oil to lightly coat. Add the scallops and cook for about 2 minutes, depending on their size and thickness, until well seared and golden. Turn the scallops over and cook for about 1 minute longer, until cooked through. Do not overcook.

Add the pasta to the boiling water and cook for 1 to 1½ minutes. Drain the pasta while still undercooked and immediately transfer to the pan containing the pepper sauce. Season

(continued)

to taste with black pepper. Bring the sauce to a boil and cook for about 2 minutes, until the sauce reduces enough to coat the pasta. Add the scallops and toss to combine.

Serve the pasta and scallops sprinkled with the chives.

JIMMY SCHMIDT
....

SWEET PEPPER, EGGPLANT, TOMATO, AND ARUGULA SANDWICH
Serves 4

Roasted vegetables turn the ordinary sandwich into something special. Jimmy likes to make his own focaccia buns, but you can use any good-quality buns for the sandwich. The toasted buns are spread with a low-calorie, low-fat mixture of mustard, papaya, and lime juice for just the right tang. Although available most of the year, papaya are at their best in the summer months. Look for yellow-skinned fruit—immature papayas are green.

1 medium eggplant, cut into ½-inch slices
Kosher salt
2 red bell peppers
2 yellow bell peppers
2 tablespoons extra-virgin olive oil
1 large Vidalia or other sweet onion, peeled and cut into ¼-inch slices
4 homemade focaccia buns (page 196) or bakery focaccia sandwich buns
¼ cup coarse-grain mustard
1 cup peeled, seeded, and diced papaya
2 tablespoons fresh lime juice
1 teaspoon freshly ground black pepper
2 tomatoes, each cut into 4 slices
About 2 ounces arugula (1 bunch), trimmed and washed

To make the filling, salt the eggplant and stand the slices upright in a colander for about 1 hour to draw the moisture out.

Roast the peppers by placing them whole on an open gas flame or outdoor grill, or under the broiler. Cook, rotating on all sides, for about 10 minutes, until the skins are black. Put the peppers in a bowl and cover with plastic wrap. Allow to cool for 15 minutes. Using your hands, peel off the charred skin. Discard the cores, stems, and seeds. Tear the peppers into large flat strips.

Prepare a charcoal, wood, or gas grill or preheat the broiler.

Rinse the eggplant under cold, running water and pat dry. Lightly brush the eggplant with about half the olive oil and grill for about 3 minutes, until lightly browned. Turn over and cook for 2 more minutes, until tender. Remove to a plate and set aside at room temperature.

Nutritional Analysis per serving (¼ teaspoon of salt added total)

Calories: 474
High in fiber and vitamins A, E, and C
Fat: 9.7 g
Saturated Fat: 1.4 g
Cholesterol: 27 mg
Sodium: 619 mg

Rub the onion slices with the remaining oil and grill for about 4 minutes, until well marked. Turn over and cook for about 3 minutes longer, until tender. Remove from the grill and allow to cool to room temperature.

Cut the focaccia buns in half lengthwise and lay cut side down on the grill. Cook for about 2 minutes, until toasted.

In a food processor, combine the mustard, papaya, lime juice, and black pepper and process to a paste.

Spread the focaccia buns with the mustard mix. Divide the eggplant slices evenly among the 4 bottom halves. Top with the red and yellow pepper slices, grilled onions, tomato slices, and finally with the arugula. Close each sandwich with the top of the buns, secure with wooden or bamboo skewers and serve.

ALICE WATERS

TOMATO CONFIT ON TOASTED BREAD WITH PESTO
Serves 4

This is a heady way to enjoy summertime's tomatoes: slow-roast them until they form a confit thick enough to spread on toasted bread drizzled with just a touch of olive oil. Top the open sandwich with pesto made with fresh, aromatic basil for a first course or a light meal. Alice prefers the texture of pesto made with a mortar and pestle, but it is acceptable to use a food processor. See the note at the end of the recipe for instructions.

Pesto
1 large clove garlic, peeled
Pinch kosher salt
1 cup finely chopped fresh basil
3 tablespoons extra-virgin olive oil
1 heaping tablespoon grated Parmesan cheese (optional)
2 grinds fresh black pepper

Tomato Confit
8 small ripe tomatoes, about 1½ inches in diameter
1 large clove garlic, peeled and sliced thin
Few sprigs fresh thyme
4 tablespoons extra-virgin olive oil
Salt
Few grinds fresh black pepper
8 slices country-style sourdough whole wheat or other full-flavored country-style bread

(continued)

To make the pesto, pound the garlic clove and a pinch of salt in a mortar with a pestle until it becomes a smooth paste. Add the basil, a few tablespoons at a time, pounding and working it into a coarse paste. As the basil mixture becomes thick and dry, add the olive oil, a little at a time. Continue grinding until the mixture becomes a thick, smooth paste and all the olive oil is absorbed. Add the cheese, if desired, and the pepper; mix well with a rubber spatula. Set aside.

To make the tomato confit, preheat the oven to 375°F.

Carefully core the tomatoes and cut each in half horizontally. Arrange them cut side down in a shallow, 1½-inch-deep ceramic gratin dish or casserole. Sprinkle the garlic slices and thyme sprigs over the tomatoes and drizzle evenly with 2 tablespoons of the olive oil. Season to taste with salt and pepper.

Bake the tomatoes, uncovered, for 1¼ hours, until they are browned, soft, and juicy. Set aside and keep warm. Do not turn off the oven.

Brush the bread with the remaining 2 tablespoons of olive oil. Lay on a baking sheet and bake for about 12 minutes, until golden brown. Cut into halves or quarters for serving, depending on the size of the slices.

Arrange the warm toasts on a platter and top with the tomatoes. Spoon the juice from the tomatoes over and around them. Spoon pesto on the tomatoes and serve immediately.

Note: Alternatively, make the pesto in a food processor fitted with the metal blade. Process the garlic and salt just until mixed. Add the basil, a few tablespoons at a time, pulsing the processor until the mixture is thick and dry. With the motor running, add the oil in a slow, steady stream until the mixture becomes a thick, smooth paste and all the oil is absorbed. Add the cheese, if desired, and the pepper and mix well with a rubber spatula.

Nutritional Analysis per serving (with cheese in pesto)

Calories: 423
Good source of fiber and vitamins A, E, and C
Fat: 26.9 g
Saturated Fat: 4.2 g
Cholesterol: 3 mg
Sodium: 484 mg

A LICE   W ATERS
....

GRILLED VEGETABLE PASTA

Serves 4

Grilled vegetables tossed with a little garlic, red wine vinegar, and basil are delicious over pasta for a quick lunch or easy supper. If you can't find every vegetable listed here, substitute another or double up the quantities of one. But don't neglect the tomatoes. They are essential to the integrity of the dish.

2 small purple eggplants, stems removed
1 small zucchini, trimmed
1 red onion, peeled
About 2 tablespoons olive oil
Kosher salt and fresh ground pepper
2 red bell peppers
2 tomatoes
1 large clove garlic, chopped fine
½ teaspoon red wine vinegar
2 tablespoons finely chopped basil
12 ounces dried fettuccine or penne

Prepare a charcoal, wood, or gas grill or preheat the broiler.

Cut the eggplant, zucchini, and onion into ½-inch-thick slices. Toss the sliced vegetables with a tablespoon of oil to coat lightly. Season with salt and pepper.

Set the bell peppers and tomatoes on the grill and then arrange the sliced vegetables around them. Grill over medium heat for 4 to 5 minutes, checking the vegetables frequently with a fork to determine tenderness and turning them so that they cook evenly and brown. The peppers' skin will char. Depending on the heat of the fire and the thickness of the vegetables, cooking times will vary. The eggplant, zucchini, and peppers may take longer to become tender than the tomatoes and onion. When fork-tender, remove the vegetables from the grill using long-handled tongs. Put the sliced vegetables in a large bowl. Peel and seed the peppers and peel the tomatoes. Chop them both coarse and add to the bowl.

Nutritional Analysis per serving (with ½ teaspoon salt added total)

Calories: 457
High in fiber and vitamins A and C
Fat: 9.9 g
Saturated Fat: 1.4 g
Cholesterol: 0 mg
Sodium: 465 mg

Add the garlic, vinegar, remaining tablespoon of olive oil, basil, and about ½ teaspoon of salt and a few grinds of pepper to the bowl. Toss the warm vegetables so that they are well coated with dressing. Set aside in a warm place.

Bring about a gallon of salted water to a boil in a large pot and cook the pasta for about 14 minutes, until cooked through but still slightly resilient. Drain the pasta and transfer to a warm shallow bowl. Spoon the vegetables over the pasta, toss well, and serve immediately.

ALICE WATERS

LITTLE MULTICOLORED PEPPER PIZZAS

Serves 4

Homemade pizzas are fun to make and taste absolutely out of this world—especially Alice's version of the American favorite, topped with a simple, colorful mixture of peppers and onions. When baking the pizzas, a layer of unglazed ceramic tiles on the floor of the oven ensures even baking. If you don't have time to make the pizza dough, you can buy it in the refrigerator section of the supermarket. However, the crust may not be as good.

Pizzas
¾ cup tepid (105° to 110°F) water
2 teaspoons active dry yeast
¼ cup rye flour
2½ tablespoons olive oil
½ teaspoon kosher salt
1¾ to 2 cups unbleached all-purpose flour

Topping
1 red bell pepper
1 yellow bell pepper
1 green bell pepper
1 Anaheim or poblano pepper, or other mildly hot pepper
1 small red onion, peeled
3 cloves garlic, peeled
½ teaspoon finely chopped fresh thyme
1 teaspoon finely chopped parsley
1 tablespoon drained capers
2 tablespoons extra-virgin olive oil, plus a little for brushing
Juice of 1 lemon
Kosher salt
Few grinds fresh pepper
5 to 6 leaves fresh basil
Grated Parmesan cheese

You don't have to, but if you decide to make your own pizza, make a sponge by combining ½ cup tepid water, the yeast, and the rye flour in a large mixing bowl and whisking until combined. Set aside for about 30 minutes to rise in a warm spot in the kitchen.

Add the remaining ¼ cup water, the olive oil, salt, and about 1½ cups of all-purpose flour. Mix with a wooden spoon until the dough begins to form a mass and comes away from the sides of the bowl. Turn it out onto a well-floured work surface and knead the dough, adding more flour as necessary to prevent sticking, for 8 to 10 minutes. When the dough is elastic, pliable, and smooth, form it into a round and dust it lightly with flour. Set the dough in a warm ceramic bowl, cover it with a kitchen towel, and set aside for about 2 hours to rise in a warm spot in the kitchen. An oven heated by a pilot light is an ideal place for dough to rise. When doubled in volume, punch down and turn out onto a lightly floured surface. Knead the dough for a few minutes, form it into a round, dust with flour and let it rise again for about 1 hour in the covered bowl set in a warm spot.

Turn the dough out onto the lightly floured work surface and divide it into 4 equal pieces. Shape these into balls and dust each one with flour. Put them on a baking sheet and cover with a cloth. Set aside in a warm spot until needed.

Preheat the oven to 450°F.

Nutritional Analysis per serving per pizza (no added salt)

Calories: 345
Moderate source of vitamins C and E and fiber
Fat: 17.7 g
Saturated Fat: 2.8 g
Cholesterol: 2 mg
Sodium: 223 mg

To make the topping, halve peppers and remove the seeds, stem, and white ribs. Slice them into thin, 1/16-inch-thick pieces. Slice the onion and garlic equally thin. Gently toss together the peppers, onion, garlic, thyme, parsley, capers, olive oil, lemon juice, and salt and pepper to taste.

Stack the basil leaves and slice them as thin as possible with a sharp knife. Set aside.

Pat each round of dough into a circle about 8 inches in diameter and about 1/4 inch thick. It might be easiest to accomplish this by sliding the dough onto your fist and turning it to make an even round. Carefully lay each mini pizza on a floured pizza paddle or inverted baking sheet.

Brush each pizza with olive oil, leaving about a 3/4-inch border. Top each pizza with an even amount of the pepper mixture so that it is about 1/2 inch thick. Bake for 15 to 20 minutes, until the vegetables are cooked and the crust is crisp, bubbly, and well browned.

Brush the edge of each pizza with a little more oil; scatter each with basil and grated cheese. Slice each into 4 or 6 slices and serve immediately.

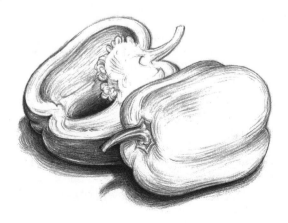

LARRY FORGIONE

BLACK BEAN SALAD WITH GRILLED CHICKEN
Serves 4

This is a wonderful combination—mildly seasoned black beans and freshly grilled chicken—but the bean salad on its own is good, too, as a side dish or meat-free meal, and a good source of fiber. You can make it ahead of time and store it, covered, in the refrigerator for two to three days. Let it come to room temperature before serving.

1 cup dried black beans
2 cups homemade chicken broth (page 193) or low-sodium canned broth,
  or water
1 teaspoon salt
1 bay leaf and 10 black peppercorns, tied in cheesecloth
1 teaspoon minced garlic
1 jalapeño pepper, cored, seeded, and diced fine
½ red onion, peeled and diced fine
2 tablespoons plus 2 teaspoons extra-virgin olive oil
2 tablespoons fresh lime juice
1 teaspoon ground cumin
1 teaspoon chili powder
3 tablespoons chopped fresh cilantro
Few drops Tabasco
Kosher salt (optional)
Few grinds fresh black pepper
4 (5-ounce) skinned, boned chicken breast halves
Lettuce leaves, for garnish
Fresh cilantro, for garnish

Put the black beans in a large pot and add enough water to cover by 2 to 3 inches. Refrigerate for 8 hours or overnight. Drain the beans in a colander and discard the soaking water. Rinse well under running water. (Or use the quick soaking method; see Note below.)

Combine the beans, chicken broth, salt, bay leaf, peppercorns, and garlic in a large saucepan. Bring to a simmer and cook for about 1½ hours, until tender but not mushy. Remove the beans from the heat and allow to cool in the cooking liquid.

Prepare a charcoal, wood, or gas grill or preheat the broiler.

When the beans are cool, drain them and discard the bay leaf and peppercorns. Put the beans in a bowl with the jalapeño, onion, 2 tablespoons olive oil, lime juice, cumin, chili powder, chopped cilantro, and Tabasco. Season the bean salad to taste with salt and pepper.

Nutritional Analysis per serving (without added salt; water used to cook beans)

Calories: 461
Excellent source of fiber
Fat: 14.9 g
Saturated Fat: 2.8 g
Cholesterol: 96 mg
Sodium: 730 mg

Season the chicken breasts with salt and pepper and brush with the remaining 2 teaspoons of olive oil. Grill for 2 to 3 minutes on each side, until cooked through.

Arrange a few lettuce leaves on each of 4 plates and spoon the black bean salad over them. Top the beans with a grilled chicken breast. Garnish each with a few sprigs of fresh cilantro before serving.

Note: To prepare the beans by the quick-soak method, put them in a large pot and add enough water to cover by 2 to 3 inches. Bring the beans and water to a boil, reduce the heat, and simmer for 2 minutes. Remove from the heat, cover, and soak for 1 hour. Drain and discard the soaking water. Rinse well. This eliminates the 8 hours of soaking.

LARRY FORGIONE
. . . .

Marinated Seafood Salad with Asparagus

Serves 4

Begin with very fresh fish for this cool, refreshing seafood salad. The fish "cooks" in the acidic marinade, becoming firm and opaque after several hours. Do not leave it in the marinade for too long or it will become mushy. Try this with warm peasant-style bread for a complete meal.

½ pound thin asparagus spears
¼ pound skinless salmon fillet
¼ pound skinless bass fillet
¼ pound small bay scallops, trimmed of small muscle attached to side
½ red bell pepper, cored, seeded, and diced fine (about ½ cup)
½ Anaheim pepper, cored, seeded, and diced fine (about ½ cup)
1 jalapeño pepper, cored, seeded, and diced fine
2 scallions, trimmed and sliced into thin rounds
½ cup fresh lime juice
1 tablespoon olive oil
3 tablespoons chopped fresh cilantro
Dash Tabasco
Few grinds fresh black pepper
Kosher salt (optional)
1 head Boston or Bibb lettuce, washed and drained

Trim the asparagus spears if necessary. Lay them in a single layer in a skillet large enough to hold them. Add water to cover and bring to a boil. Reduce the heat and simmer for 3 to 4 minutes, until crisp-tender. Carefully lift the asparagus from the pan and lay them in a shallow dish lined with a kitchen towel. Cover and chill.

(continued)

Be sure that the fish is very fresh and completely free of bones. Using a sharp knife, trim away any dark parts of the salmon and bass. Cut the fish into thin slices.

Put the fish and scallops in a nonreactive bowl. Add the diced peppers, scallions, lime juice, olive oil, and cilantro. Season to taste with Tabasco and pepper and toss gently. Cover tightly and refrigerate for 1 to 2 hours, tossing from time to time.

Season the marinated fish with a little salt. At this point it should appear to be cooked and have a firmer texture than when raw.

Season the chilled asparagus spears with a little salt and pepper.

Place a few lettuce leaves and some asparagus spears on each serving plate. Spoon the seafood salad onto the lettuce leaves and serve.

Nutritional Analysis per serving (without added salt)

Calories: 163
Good source of vitamins A, C, and E
Fat: 6.8 g
Saturated Fat: 1.0 g
Cholesterol: 44 mg
Sodium: 116 mg
Relatively low source of fiber

LARRY FORGIONE
. . . .
GRILLED NEW POTATO AND ARTICHOKE SALAD
Serves 4

Larry grills tender new potatoes, wild mushrooms, and fresh artichoke bottoms before tossing them with a simple vinaigrette and serving them over fresh garden greens for a low-fat potato salad unlike any you have tasted before.

Dressing
1 cup olive oil
1 tablespoon plus 1½ teaspoons red wine vinegar
1½ teaspoons fresh lemon juice
1 teaspoon prepared mustard
Few grinds fresh black pepper
1 tablespoon plus 1½ teaspoons chopped fresh herbs, such as chervil, tarragon, basil, or oregano

New Potato and Artichoke Salad
1 red bell pepper
6 new potatoes (about 2 pounds)
4 large artichoke bottoms (see Note)
Kosher salt (optional)
Few grinds fresh black pepper
8 shiitake or oyster mushrooms
4 cups assorted greens, such as red leaf lettuce, watercress, and arugula
2 tomatoes, seeded and diced

To make the dressing, combine all the ingredients in a small bowl and whisk together. Set aside at room temperature.

To make the salad, roast the pepper by placing it whole on an open gas flame or outdoor grill or under the broiler. Cook, rotating on all sides, for about 10 minutes, until the skin is black. Put the pepper in a bowl and cover with plastic wrap. Allow to cool for 15 minutes. Using your hands, peel off the charred skin. Discard the core, stem, and seeds. Cut the roasted pepper into strips and set aside.

Bring a saucepan of water to a boil. Cook the potatoes for about 20 minutes, until just fork tender. Drain and cool.

Prepare a charcoal or gas grill or preheat the broiler. Cut the potatoes and artichoke bottoms in half. Trim the mushrooms. Put them in a bowl and toss with 2 tablespoons of dressing. Season to taste with salt and pepper.

Grill the potatoes, artichoke bottoms, and mushrooms over medium-hot coals until lightly colored. Return the grilled vegetables to the bowl and add the pepper strips. Toss with 2 more tablespoons of dressing.

Toss the lettuces with 1 tablespoon of dressing and divide among 4 plates. Spoon the potato–artichoke salad over the lettuce, top with chopped tomatoes, and serve.

Note: For artichoke bottoms, cook the artichokes (steam, boil, microwave). When cool, peel and discard the leaves. Remove the fuzzy choke. The bottom is what remains.

Nutritional Analysis per serving (without added salt)

Calories: 292
Excellent source of fiber and vitamins A, C, and E
Fat: 14.2 g
Saturated Fat: 2.0 g
Cholesterol: 0 mg
Sodium: 173 mg

Appetizers

ALICE WATERS
....

ROCKET SALAD WITH BAKED RICOTTA
Serves 4

Nothing could be simpler and lighter than a first course of bitter greens topped with baked herbed cheese. Rocket greens are more commonly known as arugula, but also may be labeled "roquette." Buy fresh ricotta from a reputable cheese shop or specialty store—the fresher the better, especially for preparations such as this one. To save on calories and fat, you could use part-skim ricotta, but its texture may be slightly watery after it's baked.

Baked Ricotta
Nonstick vegetable oil spray
8 ounces ricotta
2 tablespoons extra-virgin olive oil
1 tablespoon finely chopped parsley
½ teaspoon finely chopped thyme leaves
½ teaspoon finely chopped summer savory or rosemary
Kosher salt (optional)
Few grinds fresh black pepper

Rocket Salad
2 teaspoons red wine vinegar
1 teaspoon balsamic vinegar
1 shallot, peeled and chopped fine
¼ cup extra-virgin olive oil
Kosher salt
Few grinds fresh black pepper
4 handfuls arugula (rocket) leaves

To bake the cheese, preheat the oven to 425°F. Lightly spray a small gratin dish with nonstick vegetable oil spray.

Mix together the cheese, 1 tablespoon of the olive oil, the herbs, and salt and pepper to taste. Spread the mixture in the gratin dish, using your fingers and a spatula to make it as even as possible. It will not be perfect. The irregular surface will turn a dappled brown in the oven.

Drizzle the remaining tablespoon of olive oil over the top of the cheese. Bake for about 25 minutes, until the top browns lightly. Remove the dish from the oven and set aside in a warm place.

To make the salad, combine the vinegars and shallot in a small glass or ceramic bowl and let stand for about 30 minutes.

Nutritional Analysis per serving (no added salt)

Calories: 295
High in vitamins A, C, and E
Fat: 26.7 g
Saturated Fat: 7.3 g
Cholesterol: 29 mg
Sodium: 70 mg
Moderate source of fiber

Add the olive oil and salt and pepper to taste, whisk until the dressing is emulsified. Set aside.

Toss the arugula with enough dressing to coat the leaves lightly and arrange the salad in high mounds in the center of each plate. Place small spoonfuls of baked cheese around and over the salad, taking care the attractive browned part shows. Serve immediately.

JIMMY SCHMIDT

SPICY SHRIMP WITH BITTER GREENS SALAD
Serves 4

Jumbo shrimp turn a simple salad into an elegant first course. These are coated with a spicy achiote paste, ground coriander (don't use fresh coriander or cilantro), and cayenne and then grilled for a spectacular presentation. The achiote paste imparts a mild, rich flavor similar to good Hungarian paprika. It is sold in Mexican and Spanish markets and specialty shops carrying a large selection of South and Central American ingredients. If you cannot find it, substitute Hungarian paprika, or make a facsimile by following Jimmy's instructions in the note below.

2 tablespoons achiote paste (see Note) or Hungarian paprika
2 tablespoons ground coriander
About 1 teaspoon ground red pepper (cayenne)
¼ cup extra-virgin olive oil
12 jumbo shrimp, shelled and deveined
2 tablespoons fresh lime juice
Kosher salt (optional)
¼ cup fresh mint leaves
1 cup flat-leaf parsley, coarse stems trimmed
½ cup fresh basil leaves
1 cup red mustard greens or other bitter greens
1 cup red leaf lettuce, torn into bite-sized pieces

Combine the achiote with the coriander, red pepper, and 2 tablespoons of the olive oil in a medium bowl. Mix to a smooth paste, adding a little cold water if the paste is too thick. Add the shrimp and toss to coat. Refrigerate for at least 1 hour and up to 2 hours.

Prepare a charcoal, wood, or gas grill or preheat the broiler.

Lift the shrimp from the spice mixture, taking care not to shake off any more of the mixture than necessary. Grill the shrimp for about 3 minutes until seared and golden. Turn and cook for about 1 minute longer until opaque. The time depends on the size of the shrimp. Lift from the grill and set aside to keep warm.

(continued)

Nutritional Analysis per serving (no salt added)

Calories: 172
Excellent source of vitamin A and good source of fiber
Good source of vitamins C and E
Fat: 14.9 g
Saturated Fat: 2 g
Cholesterol: 35 mg
Sodium: 58 mg

Meanwhile, whisk the lime juice with the remaining olive oil in a small bowl and season to taste with salt. In a medium bowl, combine the mint, parsley, basil, and both greens. Pour the lime juice dressing over the greens and toss gently.

Divide the greens among 4 plates and arrange 3 shrimp on each plate so that they stand upright and slightly overlap the greens. Serve immediately.

Note: To make a good substitute for achiote paste, mix 1 tablespoon of mild Hungarian paprika with 1 tablespoon of red bell pepper purée and 1 tablespoon of red wine vinegar. Use this for every 2 tablespoons of achiote paste.

LARRY FORGIONE
....

GRILLED SOFT-SHELL CRABS AND SWEET POTATO SALAD
Serves 4

Try this when you have the grill fired up—while it is good cooked under a broiler, grilling may provide a better flavor. The combination of soft-shell crabs and sweet potatoes gives an unexpected taste. Take care not to overcook the tender crabs—the coals should be medium hot. The crabs are most accessible early in the summer. The recipe makes more vinaigrette than you will need. Store the leftover in a tightly lidded glass jar in the refrigerator.

Vinaigrette
¼ cup red wine vinegar
½ cup vegetable oil
½ cup extra-virgin olive oil
1 clove garlic, peeled and crushed
2 teaspoons chopped fresh chives
2 teaspoons chopped fresh basil
Kosher salt to taste (optional)
Few grinds fresh black pepper

Soft-Shell Crab Salad
4 sweet potatoes, washed
8 scallions, trimmed and halved lengthwise
2 tablespoons olive oil
Kosher salt (optional)
Few grinds fresh black pepper
4 soft-shell crabs, trimmed and cleaned
4 cups assorted greens
2 tablespoons chopped parsley
1 lime, quartered

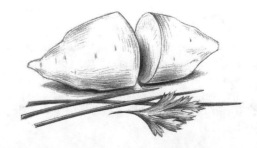

To make the vinaigrette, combine all the ingredients and whisk well. If not using right away, store in the refrigerator.

To prepare the soft-shell crab salad, preheat the oven to 350°F.

Bake the sweet potatoes for 25 to 30 minutes, until still firm and resistant. Let the potatoes cool and then slice them lengthwise into ¾-inch-long pieces. Set aside.

Prepare a charcoal, wood, or gas grill or preheat the broiler. Brush the potato pieces and the scallions with 1 tablespoon of olive oil and season to taste with salt and pepper. Grill the scallions and potatoes for 3 to 4 minutes, turning from time to time. Remove the vegetables from the grill and keep warm.

Nutritional Analysis per serving (without added salt)

Calories: 450
Great source of vitamin A
Good source of vitamins E and C and fiber
Fat: 27.4 g
Saturated Fat: 3.7 g
Cholesterol: 71 mg
Sodium: 219 mg

Brush the crabs with the remaining oil and season with salt and pepper. Grill the crabs for 2 to 3 minutes to a side, making sure the coals are not too hot and that the grill is raised high enough so that the crabs can color without burning.

Toss the greens with 2 tablespoons of the vinaigrette. Divide the salad among 4 plates and arrange the grilled vegetables on top of the greens. Set a crab on top of the vegetables, sprinkle with parsley, and garnish with a wedge of lime.

Dinner

LARRY FORGIONE

SWORDFISH WITH CHARRED TOMATO VINAIGRETTE

Serves 4

Larry recommends cooking the swordfish in a cast-iron skillet, although grilling or broiling is fine, too. He then tops the fish with a warm vinaigrette made with summer's incomparable tomatoes. This dish is relatively high in fat but low in saturated fat.

2 large vine-ripened tomatoes
¼ cup olive oil
Freshly ground black pepper
1 small onion, peeled and sliced
1 jalapeño pepper, cored, seeded, and sliced
1 clove garlic, minced
¼ cup red wine vinegar
Kosher salt (optional)
3 tablespoons chopped fresh basil
4 (6-ounce) swordfish steaks, cut at least 2 inches thick
3 tablespoons chopped parsley

(continued)

Core the tomatoes and cut them into thick slices. Brush both sides of the slices with oil and season generously with pepper.

Heat a large cast-iron or heavy-bottomed skillet over high heat until hot. Lay the tomato slices in the pan in one layer and cook for 2 to 3 minutes on each side to char. Lift the tomato slices from the pan and set aside on a plate. Repeat the procedure until all the slices have been charred.

Put the onion slices in the same pan and cook over high heat for 2 to 3 minutes, stirring, until the onions begin to brown. Add the jalapeño pepper and garlic and return the tomato slices to the pan. Cook for another 2 to 3 minutes, stirring to break up the tomatoes. Add the vinegar and 2 tablespoons of olive oil. Season with a little salt and cook for 1 minute more.

Pass the tomato mixture through a food mill to remove the seeds and skins. Add the chopped basil and keep warm.

Season the swordfish steaks with a little salt and pepper. Brush both sides of each with the remaining oil.

Heat the same or another large cast-iron or heavy-bottomed skillet over high heat until hot. Alternately, prepare a charcoal, wood, or gas grill or preheat a broiler. Cook the swordfish for 3 to 4 minutes to a side for medium. Do not overcook.

Put a swordfish steak in the center of each plate and spoon the warm tomato vinaigrette over it. Sprinkle with parsley.

Nutritional Analysis per serving (without added salt)

Calories: 343
Good source of vitamin E
Fat: 20.3 g
Saturated Fat: 3.6 g
Cholesterol: 63 mg
Sodium: 172 mg
Relatively low source of fiber

LARRY FORGIONE

GRILLED VEAL CHOPS WITH SUMMER GARDEN SALAD

Serves 4

Balmy summer days invite you outside to fire up the grill—and these veal chops, served with a simple chopped tomato salad and tender garden greens, are ideal for an easy-to-prepare supper.

1 large vine-ripened tomato, seeded and chopped
2 tablespoons chopped fresh basil
½ head radicchio, cored and chopped
2 tablespoons minced garlic
1 cucumber, peeled, halved, seeded, and chopped
1 fresh Anaheim or poblano pepper, cored, seeded, and chopped fine
2 tablespoons red wine vinegar or balsamic vinegar
2 tablespoons olive oil
Salt and freshly ground black pepper
4 (6- to 8-ounce) rib veal chops, trimmed of fat
Juice of ½ lemon
2 large handfuls tender young arugula

Prepare a charcoal, wood, or gas grill or preheat the broiler.

In a small bowl, combine the tomato, basil, radicchio, garlic, cucumber, chopped pepper, and vinegar. Add 1 tablespoon of olive oil and stir gently. Season to taste with salt and pepper. Let stand at room temperature for about 30 minutes.

Rub the chops with the remaining tablespoon of olive oil and season generously with salt and pepper.

Grill the chops for 4 to 5 minutes. Turn, and squeeze lemon juice on each chop. Cook for 4 to 5 minutes longer for medium. Cook a little longer for well done, a minute or two less for rare.

Nutritional Analysis per serving

Calories: 302
Good source of vitamins A and C
Fat: 15.6 g
Saturated Fat: 3.3 g
Cholesterol: 130 mg
Sodium: 124 mg
Relatively low source of fiber

Arrange the arugula on each of 4 plates and top with a grilled veal chop. Spoon the tomato salad over the meat and serve immediately.

LARRY FORGIONE
....

HERB-SEARED SNAPPER FILLET WITH MARINATED CUCUMBER AND TOMATOES

Serves 4

In this recipe, quickly cooked red snapper is nestled on a bed of cucumbers and surrounded by a ring of thinly sliced tomatoes for a summery presentation and full, fresh flavors. Most red snapper comes from the Gulf waters. It's a firm white fish with a fresh, mild flavor and delectable texture. Use another white-fleshed fish if you cannot find snapper—although it generally is available. Suggestions include pompano, sea bass, or mahimahi.

2 cucumbers
Kosher salt (optional)
½ teaspoon sugar
2 tablespoons red wine vinegar
4 vine-ripened tomatoes
4 (6-ounce) red snapper fillets, skinned and boned
Few grinds fresh black pepper
4 tablespoons chopped fresh herbs, such as chervil, tarragon, basil, or oregano
1 tablespoon olive oil
2 tablespoons fresh lemon juice

Peel the cucumbers and cut each in half lengthwise. Using a small spoon, scrape away the seeds. Cut the cucumbers into thin slices, put them into a nonreactive bowl, and add ½ teaspoon of salt, the sugar, and the vinegar. Toss gently and let stand for 20 to 30 minutes.

Slice each tomato as thin as possible. Arrange the slices on each of 4 plates, overlapping them to make a ring. Using a slotted spoon, remove the cucumbers from the marinade and mound them evenly in the center of the tomato rings on each plate.

Season the snapper fillets with salt and pepper. Sprinkle each fillet evenly with herbs, pressing them into the flesh with your fingers.

Nutritional Analysis per serving (no salt added)

Calories: 244
Fair source of vitamin C
Fat: 6.2 g
Saturated Fat: 1.0 g
Cholesterol: 60 mg
Sodium: 87mg
Relatively low source of fiber

Heat the olive oil in a nonstick skillet over high heat. Lay the fillets in the skillet, herb side down, and cook for 2 to 3 minutes. Lower the heat to medium-high and carefully turn the fillets over. Cook for 2 to 3 minutes longer, until the fish is cooked through.

Position a fillet on top of the cucumbers on each plate. Add the lemon juice to the hot skillet and swirl briefly. Drizzle the sauce over the fillets.

LARRY FORGIONE
....

BRAISED MAHIMAHI WITH FRESH SUCCOTASH

Serves 4

Succotash is an old-fashioned vegetable dish you may have thought went the way of great-grandma's vegetable patch and cast-iron stove. This is probably because prepared frozen succotash is a mushy, fairly unappetizing mixture. But Larry's version, made with fresh summer beans and sweet corn, is stunning—particularly when served with mild mahimahi. You may substitute monkfish, pompano, sea bass, halibut, or another white-fleshed fish for mahimahi, if necessary.

1 slice bacon, diced
2 cups shelled fresh lima beans or fava beans
1 cup shelled fresh cranberry beans or fresh peas
1 onion, diced fine (about 1 cup)
½ teaspoon minced garlic
2 cups fish broth, homemade chicken broth (pages 195 and 193), or low-sodium
    canned broth
1 bay leaf
1 teaspoon chopped fresh thyme
1 tablespoon olive oil
4 (6-ounce) pieces mahimahi, trimmed
Kosher salt (optional)
Few grinds fresh black pepper
1 cup fresh corn kernels (from 2 to 3 ears)

Cook the bacon in a large heavy saucepan over low heat just until it begins to color and the fat starts to render. Do not brown the bacon. Pour out and discard all but 1 tablespoon of fat. Add the lima beans, cranberry beans, onion, and garlic and cook over low heat for 2 to 3 minutes.

Add the broth, bay leaf, and thyme and raise the heat to a simmer. Cook for 12 to 15 minutes, until the beans are tender. Remove the pan from the heat.

Nutritional Analysis per serving (without optional salt)

Calories: 485
High in fiber
Fat: 14.2 g
Saturated Fat: 3.5 g
Cholesterol: 57 mg
Sodium: 570 mg

In another large skillet, heat the olive oil over high heat until hot. Season each piece of fish with salt and pepper. Lay the fish in the pan and brown for 1 to 2 minutes on each side.

Lift the fish from the pan and pour off the oil. Return the fish to the pan and pour the succotash over it. Add the corn, bring the succotash to a simmer and cook for 4 to 5 minutes.

Place a piece of fish in the center of each plate and spoon succotash over it.

ALICE WATERS

SUMMER MINESTRONE

Serves 4

Minestrone is a vegetable soup with pasta, beans, or rice added for substance. In Alice's summertime version, she uses freshly shelled beans, only in season for a brief time as most of the crop is set aside for dried beans. The soup also can include virtually any fresh vegetable that is in season. Check out the farmers' market or your own garden before making this luscious soup. Alice likes to add a dollop of pesto to the soup, and while it adds great flavor, it also adds calories and fat and so it is listed as optional. If you can afford the calories, please try it. Otherwise, stir a cup of finely chopped fresh basil into the soup just before serving.

1 small yellow onion, peeled
1 small leek, trimmed and thoroughly washed
1 (3-inch) piece celery
1 carrot, peeled
1 small fennel bulb, trimmed
1 tablespoon olive oil
1 cup shelled fresh fava, cranberry, or lima beans or black-eyed peas
2 tomatoes
4 cups homemade chicken broth (page 193) or low-sodium canned broth
1 cup yellow wax or green beans or *haricots verts,* or a mixture of these beans,
    topped and tailed
Kosher salt
Few grinds fresh black pepper
½ cup pesto (page 197) (optional) or 1 cup finely chopped fresh basil

Cut the onion, the white and a little of the green part of the leek, celery, carrot, and fennel into ¼-inch dice.

Heat the olive oil and 1 cup of water in a deep lidded saucepan over medium heat. Add the diced vegetables, cover, and cook gently over low heat for about 10 minutes. Add the shelled beans and cook, covered, for 20 minutes more.

Peel, seed, and dice the tomatoes, holding them over a bowl to catch the juice.

Nutritional Analysis per serving (no added salt)

Calories: 207
Excellent source of fiber and vitamin A
Fat: 5.6 g
Saturated fat: 1 g
Cholesterol: 0 mg
Sodium: 130 mg

Add the tomato juice and chicken broth to the saucepan. Return the heat to a simmer, cover, and cook for 30 minutes. Add the tomatoes and yellow or green beans and simmer uncovered for another 20 minutes.

Season to taste with salt and pepper. Ladle the soup into shallow bowls and garnish each serving with pesto, if desired, or basil. Serve immediately.

ALICE WATERS
....

BAKED SALMON
Serves 4

Baking salmon this way takes little time or effort. Be sure to buy very fresh salmon—it is practically unadorned for cooking and therefore its flavor shines as the centerpiece of the meal. Alice sets the fish on grape leaves or fig leaves, both of which impart a lovely coconutlike perfume to the fish. Grape leaves are easier to find than fig leaves—but if you can locate neither, simply bake the salmon directly on the oiled tray. Look for grape leaves in specialty markets and in stores that carry Middle Eastern food.

4 (5-ounce) salmon fillets, each about 1 inch thick
Kosher salt
Few grinds fresh black pepper
8 fresh 4-inch grape or fig leaves
About 1 tablespoon extra-virgin olive oil
½ lemon

Heat the oven to 400°F.

Season each fillet with salt and pepper and set the fillets aside at room temperature.

Wash the grape leaves and pat dry. Trim the knobby end of the stem from the leaves. Rub a few drops of olive oil on the glossy side of each leaf, spreading it evenly.

Lightly oil a baking sheet with a little more of the oil. Lay the grape leaves on the baking sheet, glossy sides up. Set a fillet in the center of a pair of leaves.

Nutritional Analysis per serving (½ teaspoon salt added total)

Calories: 244
Good source of vitamin E
Fat: 12.8 g
Saturated fat: 1.9 g
Cholesterol: 80 mg
Sodium: 290 mg
Relatively low source of fiber

Bake for 6 to 8 minutes until the leaves brown and curl a little and the salmon is just pink in the center. Remove the salmon from the leaves and discard the leaves.

Before serving, squeeze a little lemon juice and drizzle the remaining olive oil over the salmon.

ALICE WATERS
....

ROAST CHICKEN WITH ROASTED WHOLE GARLIC

Serves 4

Roasted chicken is an all-time favorite. No other preparation results in such moist, succulent meat. In this recipe, Alice flavors the chicken with lots of fresh herbs and then serves it with whole roasted garlic. During roasting, she bastes the chicken with the pan juices, and suggests using a bushy thyme or rosemary sprig to do so. You will notice that her method for roasting garlic differs somewhat from Jimmy's (see page 68). Both, however, provide tasty results.

Chicken
1 (3¾-pound) chicken
Kosher salt (optional)
Few grinds fresh black pepper
6 to 8 sprigs parsley
4 sprigs fresh thyme
1 sprig rosemary
3 cloves unpeeled garlic

Roasted Garlic
4 heads firm, unsprouted garlic
2 tablespoons extra-virgin olive oil
Kosher salt
Few grinds fresh black pepper

Trim excess fat from the chicken, being sure to check the body cavity for fat. Season the cavity with salt and pepper. Refrigerate the chicken for no more than 1 hour to give the seasonings time to mellow.

Meanwhile, prepare the roasted garlic, preheat the oven to 375°F. Rub away the loose outer skins of the whole heads of garlic to expose individual cloves. Do not separate them from the head but leave each one intact. Arrange the heads in a small ceramic baking dish so that they are closely packed. Drizzle them with olive oil and season to taste with salt and pepper. Spoon 1 teaspoon of water into the dish. Cover the dish tightly with foil and place in the oven to bake for 45 minutes. Remove the foil and bake for another 15 to 20 minutes, until the skins begin to brown and the garlic is soft with a pungent, nutty aroma. Set aside in a warm place while the chicken finishes cooking.

Nutritional Analysis per serving (no added salt)

Calories: 281
Fat: 11.9 g
Saturated fat: 2.8 g
Cholesterol: 100 mg
Sodium: 101 mg
Relatively low source of fiber

Prepare the chicken for roasting in the same oven with the garlic. Roughly chop the parsley, thyme, rosemary, and unpeeled garlic cloves and toss them together. Spoon the herbs into the body cavity of the chicken and close it by overlapping the loose folds of skin over the opening and securing them with a wooden skewer or several toothpicks. Fold the wing tips back under the wings. Season the chicken with a little more salt and pepper.

Place the chicken in a shallow roasting pan and set in the middle of the oven. Roast for about 1 hour, or until the juices run clear when tested with a fork and the thigh bone moves easily. If the bird is larger than 3¾ pounds, it may take another 15 minutes to cook thoroughly. Baste the chicken several times during roasting with the accumulated pan juices.

Remove the chicken from the oven and let it rest for about 10 minutes in a warm spot before carving. Serve the whole roasted garlic and the pan juices with the chicken. Serve the meat only and discard the chicken skin.

JIMMY SCHMIDT

Barbecued Salmon with Roasted Pepper, Sweet Onion, and Caper Salsa

Serves 4

Jimmy chooses salmon to stand up to the strong flavors of barbecue sauce and a rich roasted red pepper and sweet onion salsa. Buy your favorite smoky or hot commercial barbecue sauce.

2 red bell peppers
2 yellow bell peppers
1 Vidalia or other sweet onion, peeled and diced fine
½ cup drained small capers
¼ cup balsamic vinegar
6 tablespoons extra-virgin olive oil
Kosher salt (optional)
Few grinds fresh black pepper
¼ cup chopped fresh basil leaves
4 (6-ounce) salmon fillets
½ cup commercial tomato-based barbecue sauce
4 sprigs basil

Roast the peppers by placing them whole on an open gas flame, on an outdoor grill, or under the broiler. Cook, rotating on all sides, for about 10 minutes, until the skins are black. Put the peppers in a bowl and cover with plastic wrap. Allow to cool for 15 minutes. Using your hands, peel off the charred skin. Discard the cores, stems, and seeds. Dice the roasted peppers.

Combine the peppers, onion, capers, vinegar, and 4 tablespoons of the olive oil in a medium bowl. Add salt and black pepper to taste. Gently stir in the basil and set the salsa aside at room temperature.

Prepare a charcoal, wood, or gas grill or preheat the broiler.

Nutritional Analysis per serving (no added salt)

Calories: 489
Excellent source of vitamins A, C, and E
Fat: 31.6 g
Saturated fat: 4.5 g
Cholesterol: 90 mg
Sodium: 578 mg
Relatively low source of fiber

(continued)

Rub the salmon with the remaining 2 tablespoons of olive oil. Season with salt and pepper. Grill the salmon for about 3 minutes. Turn over and brush with a little barbecue sauce. Cook the salmon for about 3 minutes more until done. It should be firm and just beginning to flake.

Position a salmon fillet in the center of each of 4 plates. Spoon the salsa across the salmon and drizzle the remaining barbecue sauce around the salmon. Garnish with a sprig of basil and serve.

JIMMY SCHMIDT
....

GRILLED BREAST OF CHICKEN WITH SWEET CORN AND WILD MUSHROOM SALSA

Serves 4

The flavors of summer are in clear evidence in this recipe calling for roasted sweet corn and earthy chanterelles. Chanterelles, sometimes referred to as horns-of-plenty, are available from June well into the fall. Be sure to buy dry, golden specimens; avoid any that appear wet. If you cannot locate chanterelles, substitute morels, shiitake, boletes, or any wild mushroom sold by a reliable farmer or grocer.

3 large or 4 medium ears of corn, unhusked
1 large red onion, unpeeled
¼ cup extra-virgin olive oil
1 tablespoon minced garlic
2 tablespoons chopped fresh rosemary
8 to 9 ounces chanterelles or other wild mushrooms, trimmed and cleaned
3 tablespoons red wine vinegar
2 tablespoons snipped fresh chives
Kosher salt (optional)
Few grinds fresh black pepper
4 (5-ounce) boned and trimmed chicken breast halves, skin on
4 sprigs fresh rosemary

Preheat the oven to 400°F.

Lay the unhusked ears of corn in a single layer in a large roasting pan. Rub the whole onion with just enough olive oil to coat it; place in the roasting pan next to the corn. Set the pan on the bottom rack of the oven for about 30 minutes, or until the corn is tender. Remove the corn with tongs and place on a counter to cool. Continue roasting the onion for up to 30 minutes longer, until the skin is brown and the inside flesh is tender. Remove from the oven and allow to cool to room temperature. Peel to expose the tender inner flesh and dice. You should have about 1 cup of diced onion.

Husk the corn. Using a sharp knife, slice off the kernels. You should have about 1½ cups of roasted corn kernels.

Prepare a charcoal, wood, or gas grill or preheat the broiler.

Mix together the garlic, rosemary, 2 tablespoons of the olive oil, and the mushrooms in a medium bowl until the mushrooms are coated. Grill the mushrooms for about 3 minutes, turning with tongs, until golden. Return them to the bowl and let them cool. When cool, dice the mushrooms into even ½-inch pieces.

Nutritional Analysis per serving (no added salt)

Calories: 418
Good source of fiber
Fat: 18.9 g
Saturated fat: 3.2 g
Cholesterol: 96 mg
Sodium: 99 mg

Add the corn, onion, remaining olive oil, vinegar, and half the chives to the mushrooms. Season to taste with salt and pepper and set the salsa aside at room temperature.

Grill the chicken breasts, skin side down, for about 5 minutes until seared and golden. Turn and cook for about 2 minutes longer until done. Lift from the grill, discard the skins, and season to taste with salt and pepper, if necessary.

Spoon some wild mushroom and corn salsa onto the center of each of 4 plates. Slice each chicken breast on an angle into 4 or 5 slices. Lay the slices on top of the salsa. Spoon a little of the remaining salsa over the chicken and sprinkle with the remaining chives. Garnish each serving with a sprig of rosemary and serve.

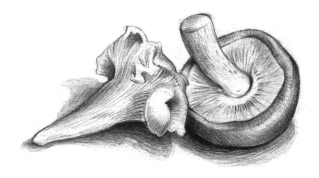

JIMMY SCHMIDT
....

CHILE-RUBBED TUNA WITH TOMATILLO CHUTNEY

Serves 4

The chipotle chiles and the tomatillo give this tuna a Southwestern flair appropriate for summertime dining. Chipotle chiles are smoked jalapeños, commonly found canned in adobo sauce. Tomatillos are sometimes called "Mexican green husk tomatoes," but although they belong to the same nightshade family, they definitely are not tomatoes. They are readily available in most groceries and certainly in those that serve a Latino population. Buy firm tomatillos with dry, light brown, papery husks. Remove the husks and wash the exposed sticky skin before dicing them.

2 tablespoons extra-virgin olive oil
1 cup diced red onion
2 cups fresh tomatillos (8 to 10 large or about 16 medium tomatillos),
    husked, washed, and diced
1 tablespoon finely diced fresh ginger
2 teaspoons ground cumin
1 cup white wine vinegar
½ cup packed light brown sugar
1 tomato, seeded and diced
2½ teaspoons puréed chipotle chiles in adobo sauce or roasted minced
    jalapeño or habañero chiles
4 (6-ounce) tuna steaks, about 1½ inches thick
1 cup fresh cilantro leaves

In a large nonreactive skillet, heat the olive oil over medium heat. Add the onion and cook for about 3 minutes, until softened. Add the tomatillos, ginger, and cumin and cook for about 10 minutes, until tender and sweet. Stir in the vinegar and sugar and cook until the sugar dissolves. Bring to a simmer and cook for about 8 minutes until the juices thicken enough to coat the back of a spoon. Add the tomato and cook for about 4 minutes, until the tomato is tender and the liquid thickens.

Remove from the heat. Add chipotle purée to taste, ½ teaspoon at a time. Set the chutney aside.

Nutritional Analysis per serving

Calories: 421
High in vitamins A and E
Fat: 16 g
Saturated fat: 3.0 g
Cholesterol: 63 mg
Sodium: 142 mg
Relatively low source of fiber

Prepare a charcoal, wood, or gas grill or preheat the broiler.

Rub each tuna steak with about 2 teaspoons of the tomatillo chutney. Grill the tuna for about 4 minutes until seared. Turn over and cook for about 1 minute for rare tuna. Cook a minute or two longer if you prefer, but do not overcook.

Put a large spoonful of the chutney in the center of each of 4 serving plates. Top with a tuna steak so that it partially overlaps the chutney. Sprinkle with cilantro and serve.

Dessert

ALICE WATERS
....

COMPOTE OF WHITE PEACHES AND NECTARINES
Serves 4

This simple, straightforward dessert calls for ripe fruit available from local orchards and green markets during summer months. The peaches and nectarines should be on the verge of turning overripe before you use them.

4 white peaches
4 nectarines
1 orange
About 1 tablespoon muscatel or sauterne (optional)
Raspberries, white grapes, or currants, for garnish

Carefully peel the peaches. Holding them over a bowl, slice them into ¼-inch-thick pieces, letting the juices fall into the bowl along with the fruit. Slice (no need to peel) the nectarines in the same way and add them to the peaches.

Squeeze the orange over the fruit. Let the fruit stand in the orange juice for about 5 minutes. Add the wine, if desired. Garnish with berries, grapes, or currants and serve immediately.

*Nutritional Analysis
per serving*

*Calories: 128
Good source of fiber
Fat: 0.8 g
Saturated fat: 0.1 g
Cholesterol: 0 mg
Sodium: < 1 mg*

ALICE WATERS
....

APRICOT SOUFFLÉ
Serves 6

It is said that a soufflé waits for no one—and this is true, once the light, airy concoction is baked. But Alice's pure-flavored apricot soufflé can be mixed up to an hour before baking, and the fruit purée, which is the base of the soufflé, can be made a day ahead of time and refrigerated. When it comes time to bake the soufflé, make sure the oven is at the correct hot temperature.

1 pound ripe apricots, pitted and quartered
About 5 tablespoons granulated sugar
⅛ teaspoon almond extract
¼ teaspoon pure vanilla extract
6 egg whites (about ¾ cup)
Confectioners' sugar, for dusting

(continued)

Put the apricots and ¼ cup of water in a nonreactive pan and cook over medium heat, stirring occasionally, until the apricots are tender. Transfer to a food processor or blender and blend until smooth. Return the purée to the saucepan and cook over medium heat until reduced to about ¾ cup. Stir in 2 tablespoons plus 1½ teaspoons of granulated sugar. Taste and add more sugar by the teaspoon, if necessary. Remove from the heat. Add the almond and vanilla extracts and stir gently. Let the purée cool.

> *Nutritional Analysis per serving*
>
> *Calories: 100*
> *Fat: 0.3 g*
> *Saturated fat: 0 g*
> *Cholesterol: 0 mg*
> *Sodium: 56 mg*
> *Relatively low source of fiber*

Preheat the oven to 425°F. Transfer the purée to a large, wide bowl.

Using an electric mixer set on medium-high speed, beat the egg whites and 2 tablespoons of sugar until foamy. Increase the speed to high and beat the whites until stiff but not dry.

Gently fold the whites into the apricot purée. Scrape the mixture into a 1-quart baking or soufflé dish or into six 4-ounce ramekins. Fill the dishes to the top.

Set the dish (or ramekins) in the upper half of the oven. Bake for 20 to 30 minutes for the large soufflé and for 7 to 8 minutes for the individual ones. When done, the soufflé will be puffed and golden brown on top. Dust lightly with confectioners' sugar and serve immediately.

Note: Once the soufflé dishes are filled with the egg mixture, they can rest at room temperature for up to an hour before baking.

LARRY FORGIONE
....

ANGEL FOOD CAKE

Serves 8

A light, airy angel food cake is one of the best desserts on a warm summer night. Serve it with fresh berries or sliced peaches.

1 cup cake flour or all-purpose flour
1 cup confectioners' sugar
2 cups egg whites (about 14 large eggs)
1½ teaspoons cream of tartar
2 teaspoons pure vanilla extract
1 cup granulated sugar

Preheat the oven to 350°F. Sift together the flour and confectioners' sugar and set aside.

Using an electric mixer set at high speed, beat the egg whites, cream of tartar, and vanilla in a large, grease-free bowl until soft peaks form. Gradually add the granulated sugar, 1 tablespoon at a time, beating until all the sugar is incorporated and the egg whites form stiff peaks. Using a rubber spatula, fold the sifted dry ingredients into the beaten egg whites, a little at a time, being careful not to overmix.

Pour the batter into an ungreased 10-inch tube pan. Bake for 40 minutes, or until the cake is firm to the touch and pulls away from the side of the pan. Remove the cake from the oven, invert the pan, and cool upside down on a wire rack for about 1½ hours. Loosen the edge of the cake with a spatula and remove from the pan. Angel food cake does not need to be cut. You can gently tear it apart with your fingers or with a fork.

> *Nutritional Analysis per serving*
>
> *Calories: 237*
> *Fat: 0.2 g*
> *Saturated fat: 0 g*
> *Cholesterol: 0 mg*
> *Sodium: 97 mg*
> *Relatively low source of fiber*

LARRY FORGIONE

Lemon Angel Food Chiffon

Serves 8

Larry starts with his angel food cake as the base for this light lemony dessert. It serves eight rather than our usual four because it is hard to cut the recipe down. Leftovers are delicious and the raspberry sauce keeps well in the refrigerator for as long as two days.

2¼ teaspoons unflavored gelatin
½ cup lemon juice
Grated zest of 1 lemon
⅓ cup plus ½ cup sugar
4 large eggs, separated
½ teaspoon cream of tartar
½ teaspoon pure vanilla extract
1 cup heavy cream, lightly whipped
Fresh raspberries, for garnish
1 (10-inch) angel food cake (page 114)

Raspberry Sauce
1½ cups fresh or frozen raspberries
½ cup sugar
1 tablespoon lemon juice

Combine the gelatin with 3 tablespoons of water in a small bowl and let soften for 2 to 3 minutes. Set the bowl of softened gelatin over warm water for 4 to 5 minutes, until the gelatin dissolves completely. Set aside in a warm place.

Combine the lemon juice, lemon zest, and ⅓ cup of the sugar in the top part of a double boiler and set it over hot water. Stir until the sugar dissolves completely. Put the egg yolks

(continued)

in a small bowl and whisk in about a third of the hot lemon juice to temper. Stir the tempered yolks into the remaining lemon juice in the double boiler.

Cook the mixture over boiling water for 4 to 5 minutes, stirring constantly, until it thickens into a custard and can coat the back of a spoon. Immediately remove the custard from the heat and stir in the dissolved gelatin.

Set the custard over a bowl of ice water and stir for about 1 minute, until slightly cooled but not cold. If the mixture becomes too cold, the gelatin will start to set and form lumps. If this happens, heat the mixture again slightly over hot water until the lumps dissolve.

Nutritional Analysis per serving (without raspberry sauce)

Calories: 474
Reasonable source of vitamin A
Fat: 13.7 g
Saturated fat: 7.6 g
Cholesterol: 147 mg
Sodium: 141 mg
Relatively low source of fiber

Using an electric mixer or a whisk, beat the egg whites with the cream of tartar until soft peaks form. Gradually add the remaining ½ cup sugar and the vanilla and whisk until firm peaks form. Fold the egg whites into the lemon custard until fully incorporated. Fold in the softly whipped cream and set aside.

Cut the angel food cake into 1- to 1½-inch cubes. You will have about 6 cups. Put the cake cubes in a bowl, add the lemon chiffon, and fold gently together. Pour the mixture into a 2½-quart loaf pan, cover, and refrigerate for at least 4 to 6 hours.

To make the raspberry sauce, put the raspberries and ¼ cup of water in a blender or food processor and purée. Pour the purée into a small saucepan and stir in the sugar and lemon juice. Bring the mixture to a simmer over low heat and cook for 2 to 3 minutes. Strain the purée through a fine strainer to remove the seeds. Cool before serving.

Dip the loaf pan in warm water to loosen the chiffon and unmold onto a serving plate. Cut into slices and serve with fresh raspberries and raspberry sauce.

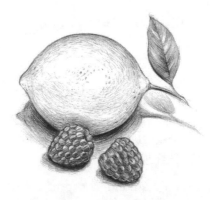

JIMMY SCHMIDT
....

NECTARINE AND BLACKBERRY CRISP
Serves 4

These individual fruit crisps are what summer is all about: fresh, ripe fruit and berries and simple preparations that don't demand much kitchen time. Make the graham cracker crumbs in the food professor or blender or put the crackers in a plastic bag and crush them with a rolling pin.

8 nectarines, sliced
1¼ cups sugar
1 teaspoon grated orange zest
1 teaspoon pure vanilla extract
1 cup graham cracker crumbs (about 12 graham crackers)
2 tablespoons unsalted butter, melted
1 teaspoon grated nutmeg
1 pint fresh blackberries, washed and hulled
Ice cream or frozen yogurt (optional)
4 sprigs fresh mint

Preheat the oven to 400°F.

Toss the nectarines with the sugar, orange zest, and vanilla extract in a medium bowl. Divide the mixture between four 12-ounce ramekins or individual soufflé dishes set on a baking sheet. Bake for 10 minutes in the center of the oven.

Meanwhile, mix together the graham cracker crumbs, melted butter, and nutmeg in another bowl. Remove the nectarines from the oven.

Nutritional Analysis per serving (without ice cream or yogurt)

Calories: 597
Good source of fiber
Fat: 10.5 g
Saturated fat: 4.8 g
Cholesterol: 16 mg
Sodium: 183 mg

Spoon the blackberries on top of the nectarines. Sprinkle the crumb topping evenly over the berries, allowing a small gap between the topping and the side of the dish.

Reduce the oven temperature to 375°F and bake for about 30 minutes longer, until the fruit is tender and the topping golden. Remove from the oven and allow to cool to room temperature on wire racks.

Serve the crisps with ice cream or frozen yogurt, if desired, and top with a sprig of mint.

AUTUMN
RECIPES

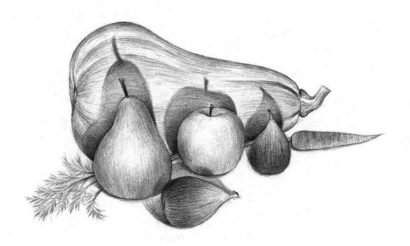

Breakfast

LARRY FORGIONE
....

WARM APPLE AND BLUEBERRY COMPOTE WITH GRANOLA AND YOGURT

Serves 4

In this recipe, Larry calls for granola—a mixture of grains primarily consisting of rolled oats but also including other grains, nuts, and dried fruit. If you have a good low-fat recipe, make your own. Otherwise, buy it from a natural foods store or a supermarket that sells a mixture that is not too high in fat. Some commercial granolas have a high fat and sugar content. Read the labels.

3 tart apples, such as Granny Smiths or Winesaps
1 pint fresh blueberries
1 tablespoon unsalted butter
2 tablespoons brown sugar
Pinch ground cinnamon
Pinch freshly grated nutmeg
1⅓ cups granola
½ cup low-fat plain yogurt

Peel and core the apples and cut them into eighths. Rinse the blueberries, discarding any that are bad and pulling off and discarding stems.

In a large nonstick skillet, melt the butter over medium heat. Add the apples and cook for 3 to 4 minutes, stirring occasionally. Add the brown sugar, cinnamon, and nutmeg and cook another minute. Add the blueberries and stir. Continue to cook, stirring occasionally, for 4 to 5 minutes, until the blueberries begin to release liquid.

Spoon the apples and blueberries into 4 serving bowls. Top each with about ⅓ cup of granola and 2 tablespoons of yogurt.

Nutritional Analysis per serving

Calories: 279
Good in fiber and high in vitamin A
Fat: 6.0 g
Saturated fat: 2.2 g
Cholesterol: 10 mg
Sodium: 117 mg

JIMMY SCHMIDT
....

APPLE AND PINEAPPLE MUFFINS

Makes 12 large muffins

Jimmy likes to make these muffins with pastry flour because it produces a finer texture. However, he realizes that not everyone has pastry flour in the cupboard all the time and suggests substituting all-purpose flour if need be. The muffins will still be great with morning fruit and a good cup of coffee. Fresh pineapple is best in the recipe, but if you prefer, use canned pineapple. Buy the kind packed in natural juices or water—not in syrup—and drain it before measuring.

3 cups pastry flour or all-purpose flour
1 cup sugar
1 teaspoon kosher salt
1 tablespoon baking powder
1 teaspoon ground cinnamon
5 egg whites, at room temperature
1 cup crushed pineapple (drained, if canned)
1 cup unsweetened applesauce
1 tablespoon pure vanilla extract
1 tart apple, cored, peeled, and diced
½ cup skim milk

Preheat the oven to 350°F. Grease and flour 12 (4-ounce) glass custard cups.

Whisk the flour with the sugar, salt, baking powder, and cinnamon.

In a mixing bowl, using an electric mixer set at medium speed, whip the egg whites until frothy. Increase the speed to high and whip until soft peaks form.

In another mixing bowl, combine the pineapple, applesauce, vanilla, diced apple, and milk. Gently fold in the egg whites.

*Nutritional Analysis
per muffin*

*Calories: 226
Fat: 2.3 g
Saturated fat: 0.4 g
Cholesterol: < 1 mg
Sodium: 258 mg
Relatively low source
of fiber*

Sift a third of the dry ingredients over the wet ingredients and fold together with a few strokes. Add the rest of the dry ingredients, about a third at a time, folding into the batter with a few swift strokes just until combined.

Spoon the batter into the cups, filling each one about two-thirds full. Set the cups on a baking sheet. Bake for 20 to 25 minutes, until golden brown and risen. The tops may crack, which is acceptable, and a toothpick inserted in the center of a muffin should come out clean. Cool slightly and then turn out of the cups onto wire racks to cool completely. Serve at room temperature.

ALICE WATERS
....

BUCKWHEAT CREPES WITH FRUIT COMPOTE

Serves 4

Alice likes to make these crepes with fresh fruit at its peak of ripeness, but you can substitute homemade or all-fruit commercial jam for the stewed fruit. Quince, apple, and pear are good choices. Heat the uncovered jar in a simmering water bath until it is fluid enough to spread easily on the crepes. The recipe makes more batter than you will need for the crepes. It keeps in the refrigerator for two days. Or make crepes using all the batter and freeze those you don't use. If separated by waxed paper and well wrapped in plastic, they will keep for a month.

⅔ cup unbleached all-purpose flour
⅓ cup buckwheat flour
Kosher salt
1¼ cups milk
3 large eggs
1 tablespoon safflower oil
2 cups chopped peeled peaches or plums or fresh berries
About 2 tablespoons granulated sugar
Confectioners' sugar, for sprinkling

In a large bowl, mix both flours with a pinch of salt. Whisk to combine thoroughly and make a well in the center of the dry ingredients.

Whisk the milk, eggs, and oil together. Pour the wet ingredients into the well in the dry ingredients and whisk thoroughly without overmixing. Strain the batter through a fine sieve into another bowl, cover with plastic wrap, and refrigerate for about 2 hours. The batter should be the consistency of heavy cream.

> *Nutritional Analysis per filled crepe*
>
> *Calories: 155*
> *Fat: 5.7 g*
> *Saturated fat: 1.2 g*
> *Cholesterol: 81 mg*
> *Sodium: 76 mg*
> *Relatively low source of fiber*

Put the fruit, ½ cup of water, and 2 tablespoons of granulated sugar in a saucepan and cook over low heat for about 10 minutes, until the fruit is soft but still juicy. If the fruit seems dry, add a little more water. Taste the fruit and add a little more sugar if necessary. Set aside and keep warm.

Preheat the oven to 375°F.

Heat an 8-inch crepe pan over medium-high heat. When it is hot, put a few drops of oil in the pan and tilt it so that the oil covers the surface. Using a small ladle, spoon about 2½ tablespoons of chilled batter into the pan and tilt it again so that the batter spreads over the surface of the pan. Set the pan on the heat and cook the crepe for about 1½ minutes, until nicely browned on one side. Turn the crepe with a spatula and cook it for about 45 seconds on the other side. Turn the crepe out onto a flat plate. Repeat with the remaining batter until you have 8 crepes stacked on the plate. Cover the crepes with a kitchen towel until ready to serve.

(continued)

Spread about 1½ tablespoons of stewed fruit on each crepe. Roll the crepes into cigar shapes or fold each into quarters. Set the crepes on an ungreased baking sheet and warm in the oven for about 4 minutes until heated through. Serve sprinkled with a little confectioners' sugar.

Lunch and Salads

LARRY FORGIONE
....

NATIVE BEAN SOUP
Serves 8

Though recipes are for four servings throughout the book, occasionally there are exceptions, as with this wonderful soup. It does not make sense to make it in a small quantity, particularly since leftovers are so good!

Posole may sound exotic but in fact it is simply dried whole corn kernels that have been boiled until soft and the husks fall off. It is very similar to hominy, a staple of Southern cooking, which is why Larry gives hominy as an alternative to posole. You can mail-order posole (from Carmen's of New Mexico, 401 Mountain Road, NW, Albuquerque, NM 87102, (505) 842-5119; Carmen's sells white and blue corn posole in 6-ounce bags) or buy it in some specialty food stores and supermarkets. Larry also calls for Jerusalem artichokes, which are also called sunflower roots and sunchokes. They are easy to find in the specialty produce section of the market or green grocer.

1⅓ cups dried posole or whole hominy (about ½ pound) or 3 (14-ounce)
    cans whole hominy, drained and rinsed
1 pound dried white beans
10 cups homemade chicken broth (see page 193), low-sodium canned broth,
    or water
2 tablespoons minced garlic (about 6 cloves)
1 cup finely chopped carrot
1 cup finely chopped onion
½ cup finely chopped Jerusalem artichokes
4 ounces smoked sausage
¼ cup snipped parsley
2 tablespoons snipped fresh sage or 1 teaspoon ground sage
1 tablespoon snipped fresh rosemary or 1 teaspoon dried rosemary
Salt (optional)
Few grinds fresh black pepper

If using dried posole or hominy, pick over and rinse it with the beans. Put both in a large bowl with about a gallon (16 cups) of cold water and let sit for 12 hours or overnight. (Or use the quick-soaking method; see Note below.) Drain and discard the liquid. If using canned hominy, soak the dried white beans only and use the canned hominy when instructed later in the recipe.

In a 6- to 8-quart Dutch oven, combine the soaked posole and beans, chicken broth or an equal quantity of water, garlic, carrot, onion, Jerusalem artichokes, sausage, parsley, sage, and rosemary. Heat over high heat until boiling. Reduce the heat and simmer, covered, for 2 hours or until the beans and posole are tender. (If using canned hominy, add it during the last 30 minutes of cooking.)

Remove the sausage and set aside to cool. Chop the sausage into bite-size pieces. Return the meat to the soup and place over medium heat until heated through. Season to taste with salt and pepper.

Note: To prepare the beans by the quick-soaking method, put the beans in a large pot and add enough water to cover by 2 to 3 inches. Bring the beans and water to a boil, reduce the heat, and simmer for 2 minutes. Remove from the heat, cover, and let stand for 1 hour. Drain and discard the soaking water. Rinse well. This eliminates the 8 hours of soaking. Do not use this method if soaking the posole with the beans.

> *Nutritional Analysis per serving (no salt added)*
>
> *Calories: 418*
> *Excellent source of fiber and vitamin A*
> *Fat: 8.2 g*
> *Saturated fat: 2.4 g*
> *Cholesterol: 10 mg*
> *Sodium: 550 mg*

LARRY FORGIONE

ROASTED CORN AND CHANTERELLE SALAD WITH AUTUMN GREENS

Serves 4

Roasting corn in the husks leaves the kernels fuller and richer tasting than usual. The corn available in the fall is more mature than the tender corn of midsummer and stands up very well to oven roasting.

3 to 4 ears corn, in the husk
About 3 tablespoons extra-virgin olive oil
6 ounces chanterelle mushrooms, trimmed and quartered
2 teaspoons minced shallots
1 clove garlic, peeled and minced
1 tablespoon cream sherry
1 tablespoon sherry wine vinegar or cider vinegar
½ teaspoon spicy brown mustard
2 teaspoons snipped parsley
½ teaspoon snipped fresh rosemary
Kosher salt
Few grinds fresh black pepper
3 cups assorted young autumn greens such as spinach, kale, mustard greens and arugula

(continued)

Preheat the oven to 350°F.

Rinse the corn and dry each ear. Rub the husks lightly with a little olive oil and arrange on a baking sheet. Bake for 15 minutes, turning once or twice. Remove from the oven and cool to room temperature. Peel off the husks and silk. With a small sharp knife, cut the kernels from the cobs and put in a bowl. You should have about 1½ cups of corn.

In a large skillet, heat 1 tablespoon of olive oil over medium-high heat. Add the mushrooms and cook, stirring, for 2 minutes, until slightly softened. Add the shallots and garlic and cook for 1 minute more. Add the sherry, raise the heat to high, and cook for about 1 minute to reduce the liquid by half.

Remove the skillet from the heat and lift the mushrooms from the pan with a slotted spoon. Add to the corn and stir gently to combine. Set aside.

Pour the liquid from the skillet into a small bowl. Add the vinegar, mustard, 1 tablespoon of olive oil, the parsley, and rosemary and whisk together to make the dressing. Season to taste with salt and pepper.

Toss the greens in a bowl with half the dressing. Spoon onto a platter. Toss the corn and mushrooms with the remaining dressing. Spoon over greens and serve.

Nutritional Analysis per serving

Calories: 184
Good source of fiber and vitamin C
Fat: 11.2 g
Saturated fat: 1.5 g
Cholesterol: 0 mg
Sodium: 32 mg

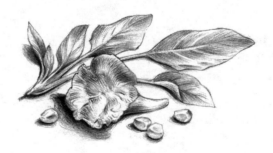

LARRY FORGIONE

PROSCIUTTO WITH A ROASTED BEET AND FIG SALAD AND A CITRUS DRESSING

Serves 4

Black Mission figs come from California, where their growing season stretches from June through November. Larry agrees with Alice that they are at their best in the fall and while he, as a New York chef, has limited access to the fragile, delicate fruit, he uses it whenever he can find fresh, ripe figs. A note of caution from the chef concerning peeling beets: Wear rubber gloves to avoid stained hands.

4 small beets
4 Black Mission figs
1 tablespoon finely chopped shallots or scallions, white part only
1 tablespoon fresh lemon juice
1 tablespoon fresh orange juice
2 tablespoons extra-virgin olive oil
Kosher salt (optional)
Few grinds fresh black pepper
2 cups frisée (curly endive), washed and trimmed
4 ounces paper-thin-sliced prosciutto
2 teaspoons snipped fresh chives

Preheat the oven to 375°F.

Wrap the washed, unpeeled beets in foil and take for 25 to 30 minutes, until tender when pierced with a fork. Unwrap the beets and set aside to cool to room temperature. At this point, turn the oven off while the beets cool or leave it on if you will be proceeding with the recipe right away.

When the beets are cool, peel them and cut them into eighths. Put the sections in an ovenproof casserole. Remove the stems of the figs and cut them into quarters. Put the figs in the dish with the beets.

Turn the oven on again to 375°F.

In a small bowl, whisk the shallots with the lemon juice, orange juice, and olive oil. Season to taste with salt and pepper. Spoon the dressing over the beets and figs.

Separate the branches of the frisée and make a nest in the center of each of 4 plates.

Arrange the sliced prosciutto around the frisée. Put the beets and figs in the oven for 1 to 2 minutes until warm.

Put 4 pieces of beet and 4 pieces of fig inside each frisée nest. Spoon the warmed vinaigrette from the casserole over the salad and prosciutto. Sprinkle with chives and serve.

Nutritional Analysis per serving (no salt added)

Calories: 210
Good source of fiber
Fat: 11.9 g
Saturated fat: 2.7 g
Cholesterol: 18 mg
Sodium: 403 mg

ALICE WATERS
....

BAKED CHANTERELLES WITH GARLIC TOASTS
Serves 4

Chanterelles are one of the treasures of the mushroom realm—golden colored, smelling of apricots (or is it peaches?), and more available than either boletes and morels, the fungi with which they are most frequently associated. Sometimes the three are referred to as a culinary trinity. West Coast chanterelles tend to be larger than those available on the East Coast, although not all specimens from the Pacific Northwest are giants. They also taste slightly different from each other, which may be caused by differences in climate and soil. Buy unblemished chanterelles, wipe them clean with a damp cloth, and slice away any dark spots on the stems or caps. Alice suggests serving these on garlic toast, but to reduce calories and fat, the baked mushrooms are delicious served on their own. Baking them *en papillote* is far easier than you might imagine and results in lovely, moist food. Cooking parchment is sold in some supermarkets and in kitchenware catalogues.

Garlic Toasts
8 (¾-inch-thick) slices baguette, cut on the bias
1 tablespoon extra-virgin olive oil
1 clove garlic, peeled and chopped fine

Baked Chanterelles
2 teaspoons extra-virgin olive oil
2 shallots, chopped fine (about 1½ tablespoons)
1 small clove garlic, peeled and chopped fine
½ teaspoon finely chopped fresh thyme
½ teaspoon finely chopped parsley
Kosher salt
Few grinds fresh pepper
Sherry wine vinegar
12 ounces chanterelles, cleaned and sliced thin

To make the garlic toasts, preheat the oven to 375°F.

Lay the bread slices in a single layer on a baking sheet. Bake for about 5 minutes until lightly toasted. Take the pan from the oven, turn the pieces of bread over, brush each with a little olive oil and sprinkle with a little garlic. Use a knife or the back of a spoon to spread the garlic evenly over the bread. Bake for about 10 minutes longer until the toasts are golden brown. Set aside in a warm place.

Raise the oven temperature to 500°F.

Heat 1 teaspoon of the olive oil and 1 tablespoon of water in a small skillet and cook the shallots and garlic over medium heat for about 30 seconds, until softened.

Remove the pan from the heat and add the remaining teaspoon of olive oil and the herbs. Season to taste with salt and pepper and a few drops of vinegar. Add the chanterelles and toss gently.

Have ready four 12 × 16-inch pieces of cooking parchment or aluminum foil. Fold a piece of parchment in half lengthwise. Open the sheet and spoon a quarter of the mushroom mixture in the center of one half of the paper. Fold the other half over the mushrooms and align the edges. Beginning at one corner (if you are right-handed, begin at the left corner facing you; if you are left-handed, begin at the right corner facing you), make tight, overlapping folds from one side across the paper to the other side so that you form a sealed half-circle. Leave about 1½ inches between the edge of the paper and the mushrooms to allow the parchment room to puff up. Seal the parchment with a secure twist at the corner. Repeat to make 4 packages.

Set a baking sheet large enough to hold the packages in the hot oven for about 5 minutes. Put the packages on the hot pan and bake for about 6 minutes until the parchment puffs up and browns.

Nutritional Analysis per serving (no salt added and without garlic toast)

Calories: 46
Fat: 2.6 g
Saturated fat: 0.4 g
Cholesterol: 0 mg
Sodium: 4 mg
Relatively low source of fiber

Nutritional Analysis per serving (no salt added)

Calories: 232
Fat: 7.7 g
Suturated fat: 1.2 g
Cholesterol: 0 mg
Sodium: 349 mg

Serve the papillotes immediately, slitting them open at the table. Pass the garlic toasts separately.

ALICE WATERS

ENDIVE, APPLE, AND WALNUT SALAD
Serves 4

This is a simple salad with very few components—but each one is in season in the fall and they blend beautifully to make an elegant salad or first course. Almost all Belgian endive actually comes from Belgium, where it is laboriously hand-grown and then shipped hours after packing. Look for slightly plump heads with yellow-tipped leaves, rather than the very thin, long heads. The bitter endive tastes best with slightly sweet apples, not any that are too tart. Alice recommends Sierra Beauties or Gravensteins.

2 tablespoons (about ¾ ounce) coarsely broken shelled walnuts
3 white Belgian endives
1 teaspoon lemon juice
2 sweet-tart apples
1 tablespoon plus 1 teaspoon extra-virgin olive oil
½ teaspoon sherry wine vinegar
Kosher salt (optional)
Few grinds fresh black pepper

(continued)

Preheat the oven to 375°F.

Spread the walnuts on a baking sheet in a single layer. Toast for 7 to 8 minutes, until fragrant, slightly browned, and crisp through-out. Transfer to another pan and set aside to cool completely.

Slice off the root end from the endives and then cut each in half lengthwise. Cut the endives into julienne by slicing them very thin with a large knife. Put the endive in a ceramic bowl and sprinkle with lemon juice. Toss gently.

Core, peel, and halve the apples. Cut each half in thin slices and then into matchstick-size julienne. Add the apples to the bowl with the endive.

Add the walnuts, olive oil, and vinegar and season to taste with salt and pepper. Toss and serve immediately.

> *Nutritional Analysis per serving (without added salt)*
>
> *Calories: 109*
> *Moderate source of fiber*
> *Fat: 7.1 g*
> *Saturated fat: 0.9 g*
> *Cholesterol: 0 mg*
> *Sodium: 11 mg*

ALICE WATERS

PROVENÇAL CHICKEN SALAD
Serves 4

This is called provençal because the peppers, olive oil, basil, capers, and anchovies are all in-tegral to the cooking of the south of France. Fennel, which physically resembles flattened celery and tastes of licorice, is more familiar in France and Italy than in the United States, al-though its popularity here is increasing every year. Look for bulbs still attached to the deli-cate fernlike leaves. Make sure the bulb is firm and white, not dry or discolored. The anchovies are optional. If you decide to use them, cut back on the salt.

½ red bell pepper, cored and seeded
½ yellow bell pepper, cored and seeded
½ red onion, peeled
½ fennel bulb, trimmed
¼ cup extra-virgin olive oil
3 tablespoons fresh lemon juice
¼ teaspoon chopped jalapeño
3 tablespoons coarsely chopped capers
2 anchovy fillets, thinly sliced crosswise (optional)
Kosher salt (optional)
Few grinds fresh black pepper
4 (4-ounce) boneless, skinless chicken breast halves
About 4 ounces frisée (curly endive)
1 cup finely sliced fresh basil

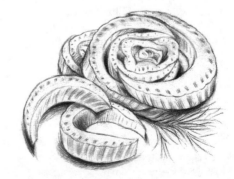

Slice the peppers, onion, and fennel into paper-thin slices.

Whisk the olive oil with the lemon juice until emulsified. Set the dressing aside.

Toss the sliced vegetables with the jalapeño, capers, and anchovies, if desired. Add the salt and season to taste with freshly ground pepper. Add the dressing and toss gently to coat. Set aside.

Prepare a charcoal, gas, or wood fire or preheat the broiler.

Season the chicken with salt and pepper. Grill for about 5 minutes on each side until the chicken is cooked through but still juicy in the center. Cool slightly and then cut the chicken into ½-inch-thick slices.

> *Nutritional Analysis per serving (without added salt and without anchovies)*
>
> *Calories: 294*
> *Moderate source of fiber and vitamins A and C*
> *Fat: 16.8 g*
> *Saturated fat: 2.7 g*
> *Cholesterol: 72 mg*
> *Sodium: 109 mg*

Add the frisée, basil and chicken to the pepper mixture and toss well. Serve immediately.

JIMMY SCHMIDT

PORK CHOPS WITH MUSTARD AND ROSEMARY
Serves 4

Spreading seared pork chops with strong mustard gives them a robust flavor that is offset by heady rosemary. Select your favorite mustard—although Jimmy recommends a bold-tasting variety rather than one that is sweet or mellow.

4 (8-ounce) loin pork chops, attached to the bone, with fat and connective tissue trimmed
Few grinds fresh black pepper
2 tablespoons extra-strong mustard
2 tablespoons coarsely chopped fresh rosemary leaves
½ cup dry white wine
4 sprigs fresh rosemary or another fresh herb, for garnish

Prepare a charcoal, wood, or gas grill or preheat the broiler. Preheat the oven to 400°F.

Season the chops with pepper. Grill for about 3 minutes until seared. Turn over and cook for about 2 minutes longer, just until seared on the other side. Transfer the chops to an ovenproof skillet or shallow baking pan.

> *Nutritional Analysis per serving*
>
> *Calories: 381*
> *Fat: 22.1 g*
> *Saturated fat: 7.5 g*
> *Cholesterol: 135 mg*
> *Sodium: 206 mg*
> *Relatively low source of fiber*

Brush the tops of the chops with mustard and sprinkle with rosemary leaves. Add the white wine to the pan. Bake for about 8 minutes (depending on thickness), until the pork chops are medium-well done.

Place the chops on a platter or 4 serving plates and spoon any pan juices over them. Garnish with rosemary and serve immediately.

JIMMY SCHMIDT

SPINACH, ROASTED PEPPER, ONION, AND MÂCHE SALAD

Serves 4

Jimmy extracts extra flavor from the onions in this recipe by first soaking them in vinegar, draining them, and using the onion-infused vinegar in the vinaigrette. Toasting the mustard seeds accentuates their flavor, too, so that this easy-to-make salad is highly flavorful. Mâche, also called lamb's lettuce or corn salad, is very mild with dark green leaves.

1 red bell pepper
1 yellow bell pepper
2 tablespoons mustard seeds
1 red onion, peeled and cut into ¼-inch slices
1 cup sherry wine vinegar
1 tablespoon coarse-grain mustard
¼ cup extra-virgin olive oil
Kosher salt (optional)
Few grinds fresh black pepper
3 cups spinach leaves, washed and patted dry
2 cups mâche leaves or red mustard greens
½ cup Italian flat-leaf parsley leaves
½ cup fresh basil leaves

Roast the peppers by placing them whole on an open gas flame or outdoor grill, or under the broiler. Cook, rotating on all sides, for about 10 minutes until the skins are black. Put the peppers in a bowl and cover with plastic wrap. Allow to cool for 15 minutes. Using your hands, peel off the charred skin. Discard the cores, stems, and seeds. Dice the roasted peppers and set aside.

Spread the mustard seeds in a small skillet. Toast them over medium-high heat for 3 to 4 minutes, shaking the pan to prevent burning, until they are fragrant and crisp. Transfer to a plate to cool and set aside.

Combine the onion slices and vinegar in a small bowl to marinate for about 15 minutes. Drain the onions and reserve 2 tablespoons of vinegar. The remaining vinegar may be refrigerated for another use; it will have a slightly oniony flavor.

Nutritional Analysis (approximately 2 tablespoons dressing per serving, no salt added)

Calories: 194
High in vitamins A, C, and E
Fat: 15.8
Saturated fat: 2.0 g
Cholesterol: 0 mg
Sodium: 91 mg
Moderate source of fiber

In another small bowl, whisk together the reserved vinegar from the onions, the mustard, and olive oil. Season the vinaigrette to taste with salt and pepper.

Combine the spinach, mâche, parsley, basil, diced roasted peppers, and onions in a large bowl. Add the vinaigrette and toss to coat the greens evenly. Serve the salad topped with mustard seeds.

Jimmy Schmidt
....

Lobster and Quinoa Risotto
Serves 4

Traditional Italian risotto is made with rice (in fact, the word *risotto* is the diminutive for *riso,* or rice), but the creamy dish, with its nearly infinite possibilities for variation, can be made with any grain that can be cooked in liquid until creamy but not mushy. Jimmy makes this one with quinoa (pronounced KEEN-wa), an ancient South American grain that is becoming increasingly popular and much touted for its health benefits. Quinoa is an excellent source of iron, calcium, vitamin E, and some B vitamins. You may have to buy it at a natural foods store, although some groceries are carrying it.

2 red bell peppers
2 (1- to 1½-pound) live lobsters
2 cups quinoa
4 cups homemade vegetable broth (page 194) or low-sodium vegetable
    broth from bouillon cubes
2 tablespoons extra-virgin olive oil
1 cup diced red onion
2 cloves garlic, peeled and minced
1 tablespoon New Mexican ground chiles or mild Hungarian paprika
Kosher salt (optional)
Freshly ground black pepper
1 cup corn kernels, cut from the cob (2 to 3 ears corn)
¼ cup chopped fresh basil
4 sprigs fresh basil or other herb

Roast the peppers by placing them whole on an open gas flame or outdoor grill, or under the broiler. Cook, rotating on all sides, for about 10 minutes until the skins are black. Put the peppers in a bowl and cover with plastic wrap. Allow to cool for 15 minutes. Using your hands, peel off the charred skin. Discard the cores, stems, and seeds. Dice the roasted peppers and set aside.

Plunge the lobsters headfirst into a large pot of boiling water and cook for 5 to 6 minutes. Transfer them to a colander and cool under cold running water. Cut the lobsters in half lengthwise and remove the meat from the tails, legs, and claws. Keep the lobster claw meat intact in large pieces and reserve for garnish. Cut the tail meat into 3 to 4 pieces each. Cover the lobster meat with plastic wrap and set aside.

Put the quinoa into a fine strainer and rinse under cold running water to remove any residue of its bitter husks. Drain thoroughly.

Nutritional Analysis per serving (no salt added)

Calories: 575
Good source of fiber and high in vitamin A
Fat: 14.6 g
Saturated fat: 2.0 g
Cholesterol: 61 mg
Sodium: 422 mg

(continued)

Bring the vegetable broth to a boil in a medium saucepan. Meanwhile, heat the olive oil in a large saucepan over medium-high heat. Add the onion and garlic and cook for 4 to 5 minutes, until tender. Add the chile powder and quinoa and cook for about 2 minutes until hot, stirring to prevent sticking.

Remove the pan from the heat and carefully pour the boiling broth over the quinoa. Return to the heat and bring to a simmer, stirring. Season to taste with salt and a generous amount of black pepper. Cook for about 8 minutes, stirring frequently, until most liquid is absorbed but the quinoa is still moist.

Add the corn, roasted peppers, and lobster to the quinoa and cook for about 3 minutes, until heated through. Add the basil and cook the risotto gently for about 2 minutes longer, until the risotto is slightly moist and creamy. Stir often.

Place a generous serving of risotto in the center of each plate. Take care to divide the lobster evenly among the plates and top each serving with a piece of claw meat. Garnish each with a sprig of basil and serve.

Appetizers

LARRY FORGIONE

MUNCHKIN PUMPKIN WITH CHANTERELLES AND LOBSTER IN A LIGHT CURRY BROTH
Serves 4

Munchkin pumpkins are mini vegetables that are widely available at farm stands and greengrocers all during the fall—particularly in the latter part of the season. Ask for small, edible pumpkins. Serve this soup with a knife, fork, and spoon, as the entire pumpkin is meant to be eaten (except for the stem!) and you will need these utensils to manage it. Even without the Munchkins, you can serve this in a bowl as you would any other soup, adding the lobster meat and mushrooms to the broth just before serving.

1 teaspoon extra-virgin olive oil
4 ounces fresh chanterelles or other wild mushrooms, cleaned and sliced
Kosher salt (optional)
Few grinds fresh black pepper
Cooked lobster meat from 2 (1-pound) lobsters, cut into ¾-inch pieces
1 teaspoon chopped fresh tarragon
4 (3-inch-wide) Munchkin pumpkins
1 teaspoon unsalted butter
½ cup finely diced carrot
½ cup finely diced leek
2 tablespoons curry powder
1 cup homemade chicken broth (page 193) or low-sodium canned broth
Chopped parsley

Heat the olive oil in a nonstick skillet over medium-high heat. Add the mushrooms and cook for 1 to 2 minutes, until slightly softened. Season to taste with salt and pepper.

Lift the mushrooms from the skillet with a slotted spoon and add to the lobster. Add the tarragon and toss gently to combine.

Wash the mini pumpkins well. Using a small sharp knife, cut a 1-inch hole in the bottom of each pumpkin. With a spoon, scrape out the seeds. Season the inside of each pumpkin with salt and pepper. Put the pumpkins in a steaming basket set in a deep saucepan over about an inch of water, cover, and steam for 18 to 20 minutes, until tender. Remove from the steaming basket and set aside to cool. (Do not dismantle the steamer.)

> *Nutritional Analysis per serving*
>
> *Calories: 295*
> *Fat: 4.5 g*
> *Saturated fat: 1.2 g*
> *Cholesterol: 165 mg*
> *Excellent source of vitamin A*
> *Moderate source of fiber and good source of vitamin E*
> *Sodium: 1,067 mg*

Fill each pumpkin with the lobster and chanterelle mixture, pressing firmly with your fingers to keep the stuffing in place.

In a small saucepan, combine the butter, carrot, leek, and curry powder. Cook over low heat, stirring, for 2 to 3 minutes. Add the broth and bring to a simmer. Simmer for 2 to 3 minutes. Keep hot.

Return the stuffed pumpkins to the steaming basket and add more water, if necessary. Steam for 3 to 4 minutes until heated through.

Put a steamed pumpkin in the center of each of 4 shallow soup dishes and ladle the curry broth around it. Sprinkle with parsley and serve.

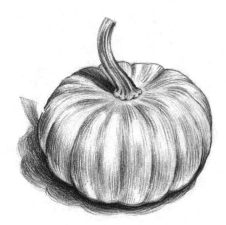

JIMMY SCHMIDT
....

GRILLED WILD MUSHROOMS WITH PARSLEY AND GARLIC VINAIGRETTE

Serves 4

Few first courses are as easy to prepare as this one with grilled forest mushrooms. The fire should be hot, but make sure the grid is not too close to the coals so that the mushrooms turn golden and don't char. You can, of course, broil the mushrooms under the broiler but the flavor imparted by grilling is probably going to be better.

3 tablespoons balsamic vinegar
6 tablespoons extra-virgin olive oil
1½ cups plus 2 tablespoons chopped Italian flat-leaf parsley
2 tablespoons grated lemon zest
1 anchovy fillet, mashed into a paste (optional)
4 cloves garlic, peeled, minced fine, and separated
Kosher salt (optional)
Freshly ground black pepper
1½ pounds wild mushrooms, preferably chanterelle, portobello, or shiitake,
    cleaned and stemmed

Prepare a charcoal, wood, or gas grill or preheat the broiler.

Combine the vinegar, 3 tablespoons of the olive oil, 2 tablespoons of chopped parsley, the lemon zest, anchovy, and 1 of the minced garlic cloves in a small bowl. Mix well. Season to taste with salt and a generous amount of black pepper. Set the vinaigrette aside.

Combine the remaining 3 tablespoons of olive oil and the garlic and toss with the mushrooms. Season to taste with black pepper.

Grill the mushrooms for 2 to 3 minutes, depending on their size, until golden. Turn the mushrooms over and grill for about 1 to 2 minutes longer until they are evenly cooked. Alternatively, broil the mushrooms about 4 inches from the heat.

Return the mushrooms to the bowl and toss with the 1½ cups of parsley. Divide the mushrooms and parsley among 4 plates. Whisk the vinaigrette and drizzle it over the mushrooms. Sprinkle a little black pepper over the plates and serve.

Nutritional Analysis per serving (no salt added; no anchovies)

Calories: 239
Fat: 21.3 g
Saturated fat: 2.9 g
Cholesterol: < 1 mg
Moderate source of fiber and vitamin C
Sodium: 49 mg

ALICE WATERS
....

MARINATED SARDINE FILLETS

Serves 4

You may not be used to the idea of sardines that are not packed in cans, but fresh sardines are available through good fishmongers and well worth a search. In Europe, they are more abundant than here, and they are also more easily found near West Coast waters than East Coast. Sardines are immature pilchards, members of the herring family. You can substitute fresh herring for sardines in this recipe. Whether you get sardines or herring, ask the fish merchant to fillet them for you—or follow Alice's instructions. Although the sardines are not "cooked" with heat, they are cured in salt—with delicious results.

8 (8-ounce) whole fresh sardines
1 tablespoon kosher salt
Juice of 1 lemon
2 tablespoons extra-virgin olive oil
1 tablespoon minced parsley

If sardines or herring are not filleted:

Using a very sharp small knife, remove a fillet from a sardine by running the knife the length of the spine, from head to tail. Carefully remove the intact fillet from the fish, leaving no excess on the bone. Repeat on the other side so that each fish yields 2 fillets. Discard the head, bones, and tail.

Remove the tiny bones along the midline of each fillet by making an incision that goes nearly the length of the fillet. Discard the bones and lay the fillets, flesh side up, on a large platter.

Nutritional Analysis per serving

Calories: 154
Fat: 12 g
Saturated fat: 2.1 g
Relatively low source of fiber
Sodium: 1,400 mg
Cholesterol: 35 mg

Sprinkle the fillets with half the salt. Turn them over and sprinkle with the remaining salt. Cover tightly with plastic wrap and refrigerate for at least 3 hours to cure them. If the fillets are more than ½ inch thick, let them cure for 4 hours.

Serve the fillets, 4 to a person, drizzled with lemon juice and olive oil and sprinkled with parsley.

Dinner

ALICE WATERS
....

GRILLED STEAK WITH GREMOLATA

Serves 4

This recipe is an example of how red meat, in this instance steak, can be part of a low-calorie, low-fat diet. While Alice does not advocate eating red meat often, it is delicious every now and then. These fillets are rubbed with salt and pepper about an hour before they are grilled and then are served on wilted greens. Easy. Excellent. And they are not too high in fat or cholesterol.

4 (6-ounce) fillet steaks, each about 1¼ inches thick
Kosher salt
4 teaspoons coarsely ground fresh pepper
3 tablespoons finely chopped parsley
½ teaspoon finely chopped garlic
⅓ teaspoon finely chopped lemon zest
About 4 ounces frisée (curly endive)
Few grinds fresh black pepper

About 1 hour before cooking, rub the fillets with a little salt and the coarsely ground pepper. Press the pepper into the meat so that it adheres. Let the meat sit at cool room temperature for about 1 hour.

Combine the parsley, garlic, and lemon zest in a small bowl to make the gremolata.

Prepare a charcoal, wood, or gas grill, or preheat the broiler. Grill the fillets for 5 to 6 minutes on each side for medium rare. They should spring back slightly when pressed in the center. Set aside in a warm place.

Nutritional Analysis per serving

Calories: 281
Fat: 12.9 g
Saturated fat: 4.8 g
Cholesterol: 107 mg
Relatively low source of fiber
Sodium: 313 mg

Heat 1 tablespoon of water with a little salt and the pepper in a small stainless steel pan. Add the frisée and cook, turning with tongs, for about 1 minute, until the frisée wilts. Lift the frisée from the pan, shake, and transfer to a serving platter. Spread the wilted frisée over the platter and top with the fillets. Sprinkle the steaks with the gremolata and serve.

ALICE WATERS
....
PASTA WITH CLAMS, THYME, AND GARLIC
Serves 4

Pasta with clam sauce is almost a classic. Alice Waters' version relies on fresh littlenecks, fresh thyme, and fresh pasta. Littlenecks are the smallest size of quahogs: hard-shell clams from the Atlantic Coast. Cherrystones are a little bigger than littlenecks, and when quahogs grow to be more than three inches in diameter, they become chowder clams. Littlenecks are small, tender, and wonderfully sweet. Buy them in the shell to ensure freshness; you will also need their cooking liquid for the sauce. Be sure to strain it well.

4 pounds littleneck clams, in the shell
1 cup diced onion
1 clove garlic, crushed but intact
2 to 3 sprigs fresh thyme
2 bay leaves
Few grinds fresh black pepper
½ cup white wine
2 tablespoons finely chopped parsley
1 teaspoon finely chopped fresh thyme
2 cloves garlic, chopped fine
¼ teaspoon finely chopped lemon zest
12 ounces fresh tagliatelle or linguine
2 tablespoons extra-virgin olive oil
Juice of ½ lemon

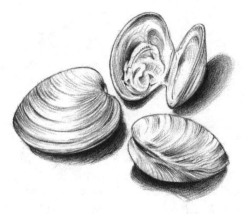

Rinse the clams under cold running water. Put the clams, onion, crushed garlic, thyme sprigs, bay leaves, pepper, and white wine in a stainless steel saucepan with a tight-fitting lid. Bring to a simmer, cover, and steam for 4 to 5 minutes until the clams open. Remove the clams from the broth and let them cool. Discard any clams that do not open. Set aside the broth.

Nutritional Analysis per serving

Calories: 480
Fat: 9.7 g
Saturated fat: 1.3 g
Cholesterol: 48 mg
Good source of fiber
Sodium: 87 mg

Shuck the clams over a bowl to catch any released juices. Set aside the shucked clams and add the juices to the reserved broth. Strain the broth through a fine sieve or a double thickness of cheesecloth. Taste for saltiness; if too salty, remove a tablespoon or so and replace it with water or fish broth. Set aside.

Combine the chopped parsley, thyme, chopped garlic, and lemon zest in a small bowl to make gremolata. Set aside.

Bring about a gallon of salted water to a boil and add the pasta. Cook for 1½ to 2 minutes until the pasta is firm and resilient. Drain.

Meanwhile, bring the clam broth to a simmer and add the shucked clams, olive oil, and lemon juice. Immediately remove the pan from the heat. Toss the clams and broth with the hot pasta. Add the gremolata and toss again. Transfer to a warm bowl and serve immediately.

ALICE WATERS
....

ONION AND ROASTED PEPPER PANADE
Serves 4

For this simple, country-style dish, Alice roasts peppers that have been sliced and seeded before being put in the oven—a method similar to roasting whole peppers that brings out the incomparable sweetness of vine-ripened red bell peppers. She combines the peppers with caramelized onions and slices of rustic bread. The fat content is raised because of the Parmesan cheese, which you could reduce if you prefer.

2 tablespoons olive oil
3 large onions, peeled and sliced thin
4 large red bell peppers, halved, cored, and seeded
8 large slices country-style whole wheat sourdough bread, lightly toasted
Kosher salt (optional) and a few grinds of fresh black pepper
4 cups homemade chicken broth (page 193) or low-sodium canned broth
¼ cup grated Parmesan cheese

Preheat the oven to 375° F.

Heat the olive oil in a large skillet over medium heat. Add the onions, lower the heat, and cook gently for about 35 minutes, until caramelized. Scrape the bottom of the pan several times during cooking to prevent sticking and to incorporate any brown bits with the onions. When golden brown, set aside.

Meanwhile, lay the peppers, skin side up, in a single layer in a shallow roasting pan. Roast for 35 to 40 minutes, until the skins are brown and the flesh is soft. Let the peppers cool slightly and then peel off the skin and slice the peppers into ¼-inch strips.

> *Nutritional Analysis per serving (without added salt)*
>
> *Calories: 208*
> *Fat: 7.2 g*
> *Saturated fat: 1.7 g*
> *Cholesterol: 3 mg*
> *Good source of fiber and vitamins A and C*
> *Sodium: 533 mg*

Lay 4 slices of toast in a 3-inch-deep baking pan large enough to hold the bread in a single layer. Spread a quarter of the onions over the bread and season lightly with salt and pepper. Spread half the roasted peppers over the onions and season lightly again. Top with another quarter of the onions and the rest of the peppers, seasoning lightly with salt and pepper. Lay the remaining 4 slices of toast over the vegetables.

Pour about half the chicken broth into the pan so that it comes just to the top of the toast. Sprinkle with cheese.

Cover the baking pan tightly with foil, set in the center of the oven, bake for about 45 minutes until the top is crisp.

Combine the rest of the onions and broth in a saucepan and bring to a simmer. Cut the baked panade into quarters and put in shallow soup bowls. Ladle about ½ cup of broth over the panade in each bowl and serve.

JIMMY SCHMIDT
....

BREAST OF PHEASANT OR CHICKEN WITH PUMPKIN AND CRANBERRIES

Serves 4

Munchkin pumpkins and Golden Babies pumpkins are sold in farm markets and groceries in the fall when all squash are at their peak. You can, in a pinch, use the flesh from sugar pumpkins (the kind used to make pumpkin pie) or even unsweetened canned pumpkin purée, but neither the flavor nor the presentation will be as nice. And there will be no pumpkin shell to put on the plates. (Be sure you don't use a small jack-o'-lantern pumpkin.) Jimmy designed this dish to take advantage of the wonderful flavors of fall, which often include game birds. If you prefer, however, use boneless chicken breasts in place of pheasant.

10 Munchkin or Golden Babies pumpkins
8 large shallots, skin on
Kosher salt (optional)
Few grinds fresh black pepper
½ pound cranberries, washed and stemmed
½ cup sugar
½ cup dry red wine
4 cups homemade vegetable broth (page 194) or low-sodium vegetable
    broth from bouillon cubes
¼ cup snipped fresh chives
4 (6-ounce) boneless pheasant breasts or chicken breast halves
4 chives or sprigs of other herbs, for garnish

Preheat the oven to 375° F.

Carefully cut the tops off the pumpkins or squash; scoop out the seeds and discard them. Set the pumpkins upright in an ovenproof baking dish just large enough to hold them snugly. Set the lids back on the pumpkins. Add the unskinned shallots to the dish and place on the lower rack of the oven. Cook for about 1 hour and 20 minutes, until the pumpkins are tender. Check the shallots after about 1 hour; if they are very soft and tender, remove them from the oven. When the pumpkins are tender, remove them from the oven and lower the oven temperature to 200° F.

Scoop the pumpkin flesh from the shells. Reserve the 4 best shells. Peel the shallots, dice them fine, and mix them with the pumpkin flesh. Season to taste with salt and pepper. Keep the pumpkin mixture and shells warm in the oven.

Meanwhile, combine the cranberries, sugar, and ½ cup of water in a medium saucepan. Bring to a simmer over medium-high heat and cook for about 5 minutes, until the cranberries burst. Using a slotted spoon, remove ½ cup of whole cranberries from the pan.

Nutritional Analysis per serving (no salt added)

Calories: 433
Fat: 7.2 g
Saturated fat: 2.3 g
Cholesterol: 98 mg
Moderate source of fiber and a good source of vitamin C
Excellent source of vitamin A
Sodium: 135 mg

(continued)

Take the pumpkin mixture from the oven and carefully fold the ½ cup of cranberries into the warm pumpkin. Return the pumpkin mixture to the oven and keep warm.

Continue cooking the remaining cranberries for about 5 minutes until they are very soft. Transfer the cranberries and their liquid to a blender or food processor, add the red wine, and carefully purée until smooth. Strain through a fine sieve to remove the skins and seeds. Add a little more wine if necessary to keep the sauce consistency pourable. Keep warm.

In another medium saucepan, bring the vegetable broth to a simmer over high heat and cook for about 12 minutes, until reduced to ½ cup. Season to taste with salt and pepper. Add the chives and keep warm.

Prepare a charcoal, wood, or gas grill or preheat the broiler.

Lay the pheasant or chicken breasts on the grill or under the broiler, skin side toward the heat, and cook for about 4 minutes, until well seared and golden. Turn over and cook for about 3 more minutes, depending on the thickness of the breasts. Remove and discard the skin.

Take the 4 warm pumpkin shells from the oven and fill each generously with the hot pumpkin-cranberry mixture. Set the pumpkin lids on each. Place a filled pumpkin on each of 4 serving plates and spoon the remaining mixture next to the shells. Drizzle the cranberry sauce lightly over the pumpkin mixture and across the plate. Cut each pheasant breast into 4 or 5 thin slices lengthwise and fan, slightly overlapping the pumpkin mixture, in the center of the plates. Spoon the chive sauce over the pheasant and pumpkin. Garnish each plate with a few chives inserted into the pumpkin mixture.

JIMMY SCHMIDT
. . . .

DUCK WITH DRIED CHERRIES AND SAGE, MASHED PARSNIPS AND POTATOES

Serves 4

Seared duck breasts taste very good with fruity sauces, such as this one made with dried tart cherries. Dried cherries are sold in most specialty shops and are beginning to show up in supermarkets, too. All dried cherries used to be tart, but some growers are now marketing dried sweet cherries, so be sure to check the packaging. You could also substitute raisins or currants, if necessary.

To save on calories and fat in this dish, omit the fried sage and sage oil. Replace the oil in the parsnips and potatoes with a little more cooking liquid. Replace the fried sage with about half the amount (two tablespoons) of fresh leaves, sliced into julienne and scattered over the dish just before serving. Both measures will shrink the calorie count to 196 per serving and the fat to 7.2 grams.

8 ounces pearl onions or shallots, unpeeled
1 cup dried tart cherries
¼ cup red wine vinegar
2 cups homemade vegetable broth (page 194) or low-sodium vegetable broth
  from bouillon cubes
1 cup dry red wine, such as Pinot Noir
Kosher salt
Freshly ground black pepper
1 baking potato, peeled and cut into large chunks
4 large parsnips, peeled and cut into large chunks
¼ cup extra-virgin olive oil
¼ cup fresh sage leaves plus 4 sprigs fresh sage
4 (6- to 7-ounce) boneless duck breasts, skinned and trimmed of all fat

Preheat the oven to 400° F.

Put the onions in a small ovenproof baking dish, cover, and bake for about 1 hour until very tender. Cool to room temperature and carefully peel, taking care that they retain their shape. Set aside.

Combine the cherries, vinegar, wine, and broth in a large saucepan and bring to a simmer over medium-high heat. Cook for about 15 minutes, until the liquid has thickened enough to coat the back of a spoon. Season to taste with salt and pepper. Add the onions and keep warm.

Put the potato and parsnip chunks into a large pot and cover with water. Bring to a simmer over medium heat and cook for 15 to 20 minutes, until very tender. Remove from the heat and let the vegetables sit in the hot liquid for about 3 minutes.

Meanwhile, pour the oil into a small saucepan and heat to 300° F. Add the ¼ cup of sage leaves and cook for about 3 minutes, until crisp. Using a slotted spoon, carefully lift the sage from the oil and drain on a paper towel. Reserve the oil.

Drain the potato and parsnip chunks in a colander over another pot or bowl to collect the cooking liquid. Transfer the vegetables to a large bowl, add the 2 tablespoons of reserved sage oil, and mash with a fork or potato masher or whip with a hand-held electric mixer until smooth. If the consistency is too thick, add a little of the cooking liquid. Season to taste with salt and a generous amount of black pepper and set aside.

Cook the duck in a skillet, skin side down, for about 4 minutes, until well seared. Turn over and cook for about 3 minutes more, depending on the thickness of the breasts, until done.

Spoon the mashed parsnips and potatoes onto the upper third of each of 4 serving plates. Cut each duck breast into 4 to 5 slices lengthwise and fan them across the plates, overlapping the mashed vegetables slightly. Spoon the cherry sauce around each plate and lightly drizzle it over the duck. Sprinkle the sage leaves over the mashed vegetables and serve.

Nutritional Analysis per serving

Calories: 476
Fat: 18.7 g
Saturated fat: 4.9 g
Cholesterol: 113 mg
Excellent source of fiber and vitamin A
Good source of Vitamins C and E
Sodium: 395 mg

Nutritional Analysis per serving (potatoes and parsnips only; without added salt)

Calories: 250
Fat: 13.9 g
Saturated fat: 2 g
Cholesterol: 0 mg
High in fiber
Sodium: 15 mg

Jimmy Schmidt
....

Grilled Salmon with Apples and Juniper

Serves 4

Jimmy makes a sauce for the salmon with pomegranate juice, apples, onions, and juniper berries (you need only twelve of these potent berries to flavor the sauce), all of which capture
many of the flavors of fall. Pomegranates are at their peak in late October and November,
and since their season is so brief, those who appreciate the sweet-tart fruit with its ruby-red,
juicy seeds are always looking for ways to utilize them. Here's a wonderful idea.

1 large pomegranate
2 cups apple cider
2 cups homemade fish broth (page 195) or water
½ cup cider vinegar
12 juniper berries
1 tablespoon fresh thyme leaves
1 tablespoon whole black peppercorns
1 small red onion, peeled and diced fine
Kosher salt (optional)
Few grinds fresh black pepper
½ cup finely diced green apple, preferably Rhode Island Greening or
    Granny Smith, skin on
4 (5-ounce) skinless, boneless salmon fillets
¼ cup snipped fresh chives
Fresh chives or parsley, for garnish

Prepare a charcoal, wood, or gas grill or preheat the broiler.

Cut the pomegranate in half. Pick up one half with both hands and
hold it over a plate, cut side down. Press your thumbs together at
one end and apply pressure while pulling the skin back with your
fingers to turn the pomegranate inside out. This will release the
seeds and membrane. Carefully separate the seeds from the membrane and set them aside. Using a citrus juicer, squeeze the juice
from the other half of the pomegranate. Discard all rind and
membrane.

*Nutritional Analysis
per serving (without
added salt)*

*Calories: 317
Fat: 9.6 g
saturated fat: 1.52 g
Cholesterol: 80 mg
Moderate source of
fiber
Sodium: 69 mg*

Combine the cider, fish broth, vinegar, juniper berries, thyme, peppercorns, and pomegranate juice in a medium nonreactive saucepan. Bring to a boil over medium heat and boil for about 10 minutes, until reduced to 1¼ cups. Strain through a fine
sieve.

Put the onion in a large nonstick skillet, cover, and cook over medium-high heat for about
5 minutes until the onion begins to soften. Add the reduced broth and cook for about 3
minutes, until the onion is tender. Season to taste with salt and pepper. Add the apple and
cook for about 2 minutes, until the apple is still slightly firm when bitten into. Keep warm.

Grill or broil the salmon with the inside flesh toward the heat source for about 4 minutes, until well seared. Turn over and cook for about 2 minutes longer, depending on the thickness of the salmon.

Spoon half the sauce over 4 serving plates. Set a salmon fillet in the center of each plate. Add the chives to the remaining sauce and spoon it over the tops of the salmon fillets. Sprinkle the reserved pomegranate seeds around the salmon on the plate. Garnish with chives and serve.

LARRY FORGIONE

ROAST CHICKEN WITH APPLE-SAGE DRESSING

Serves 4

Larry first developed this recipe using pheasant, but since more people cook chicken than pheasant, he revised it. He strongly urges home cooks to buy free-range chickens, which taste significantly better than supermarket varieties, have less fat and are usually raised without antibiotics. The dressing is not meant to be stuffed into the chicken but instead is baked in a casserole and served on the side. It can also be made a day ahead of time and reheated for about 45 minutes until hot.

The sauce for the chicken requires that you peel small onions, a tricky task unless you first immerse the whole onions in boiling water for 3 minutes, drain, trim the root ends and then gently press them to slip out of the skins. If you prefer, you can substitute dried chestnuts for roasted. Simmer 1½ ounces (about ⅓ cup) of dried chestnuts in water, covered, for 1½ to 2 hours until they are completely rehydrated. Drain and proceed with the recipe. By the way, if you choose to substitute pheasant for chicken in the recipe, the chef recommends discarding the pheasant legs after cooking as the meat is tough and stringy.

Apple-Sage Dressing
1 tablespoon extra-virgin olive oil
1½ teaspoons lightly salted butter
¾ cup cubed tart apple (1 large apple)
2 tablespoons chopped fresh sage leaves
½ teaspoon minced garlic
⅓ cup finely chopped onion
¾ cup homemade chicken broth (page 193) or low-sodium canned broth
4 cups cubed dried bread (7 to 8 slices)
Pinch kosher salt (optional)
⅛ teaspoon freshly ground black pepper

(continued)

Chicken
2 (2-pound) chickens
Extra-virgin olive oil
Kosher salt (optional)
Few grinds fresh black pepper
1 onion, peeled and sliced
1 tart apple, cored and sliced
1 clove garlic, peeled and minced
1½ cups homemade chicken broth or low-sodium canned broth
1½ teaspoons cornstarch
½ cup heavy cream
½ cup peeled cooked chestnuts, chopped
2 tablespoons applejack (apple brandy)
3 cups small boiling onions, peeled (about 36 onions)
¼ cup sugar
¼ cup unsalted butter
Freshly snipped chives

To make the apple-sage dressing, preheat the oven to 375° F.

In a large skillet, heat the olive oil and butter. Add the apple, sage, garlic, and onion. Cook, stirring, for about 2 minutes. Carefully add the broth and cook for 1 minute more.

Put the bread cubes in a large mixing bowl. Pour the broth mixture over the bread. Toss to moisten evenly. Season with salt and pepper. Spoon the mixture into a 1½-quart casserole. Bake uncovered for 20 to 25 minutes, or until heated through. You may cook the stuffing in the oven with the chicken. Time it so that you put the stuffing in the oven about 20 minutes before the chicken is done.

Nutritional Analysis per serving (without skin)

Calories: 858
Fat: 43.9 g
Saturated fat: 19.3 g
Cholesterol: 171 mg
Sodium: 663 mg
High in vitamin A and fiber

To prepare the chickens, remove the liver and giblets from the cavities, if necessary, and reserve for another use. Remove and coarsely chop the wings and neck. Tie the legs securely to the tail. Rub the chickens with olive oil and season to taste with salt and pepper.

Pour 2 tablespoons of olive oil into a large roasting pan and put the roasting pan in the oven for 2 minutes. Lay the chickens on one side in the pan and roast for 15 minutes. Turn them onto the other side and roast for 15 minutes more.

Remove the chickens from the oven and spoon off the fat in the pan. Turn the chickens breast side up. Add the chopped wings, necks, onion, apple, and garlic to the pan. Roast for 30 to 40 minutes, stirring the vegetable mixture once or twice, until a leg joint moves easily and the juices run clear when a thigh is pricked with a knife. Remove the chickens from the pan and cover with foil to keep warm.

Pour off as much fat as possible from the pan. Stir the chicken broth into the pan drippings, scraping up browned bits as you do. Strain the broth into a measuring cup, discard the solids, and skim off the fat. Transfer the broth to a saucepan and bring to a boil. Cook, uncovered, over medium-high heat for 8 to 10 minutes or until reduced to about ½ cup.

In a small bowl, stir together the cornstarch and 1 tablespoon of the cream. Stir the remaining cream into the broth and then add the cornstarch-cream mixture to the broth. Cook, stirring, for 3 to 4 minutes over medium-high heat until thickened and bubbly. Reduce the heat to medium and cook for another 2 minutes, stirring. Stir in the chestnuts and applejack and heat thoroughly. Set aside to keep warm.

Meanwhile, put the onions, sugar, butter and 1½ cups of water into a 10-inch skillet. Cook, uncovered, over high heat for 15 to 20 minutes, or until the mixture is golden and the onions are caramelized, stirring occasionally. Remove with a slotted spoon and keep warm.

Remove the meat from the thighs, legs, and breasts. To serve, put a large spoonful of Apple-Sage Dressing in the center of each plate. Arrange some meat on each plate. Spoon chestnut sauce over the meat and dressing and surround with caramelized onions. Sprinkle with chives.

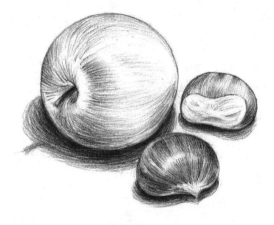

LARRY FORGIONE
....

VENISON POT ROAST WITH ROOT VEGETABLES AND PARSNIP WHIPPED POTATOES

Serves 4

Venison is a wonderful meat that is a relatively low-fat alternative to beef. Larry likes to cook with it whenever possible and finds that his customers enjoy it. You can probably buy venison through your butcher or mail order it from specialty food companies (see Note). If you prefer, substitute brisket or top round. Omit the bacon if you use beef. It's interesting to compare Larry's and Jimmy's recipes for mashed parsnips and potatoes. (Jimmy's is on page 142). Both are delicious.

Pot Roast
2 slices bacon
2 teaspoons extra-virgin olive oil
1 (1½-pound) rolled and tied leg of venison or (2-pound) fresh beef brisket
    or boneless beef top round
⅔ cup beef broth
2 tablespoons dry red wine
Kosher salt (optional)
Few grinds fresh black pepper
5 to 6 sprigs fresh thyme
6 small whole onions, peeled
¼ pound rutabaga, peeled and cut into 1-inch cubes
1 medium turnip, peeled and cut into eighths
1 large carrot, peeled and cut into 1½-inch lengths
2 cloves garlic, peeled and cracked (crushed but left whole)
2 teaspoons unsalted butter, softened
2 teaspoons cornstarch
1 tablespoon chopped Italian flat-leaf parsley
1 teaspoon minced fresh thyme leaves

Parsnip Whipped Potatoes
1½ pounds potatoes (about 3 potatoes), peeled and cut into 1-inch cubes
1 pound parsnips (about 3 parsnips), peeled and cut into 1-inch pieces
Kosher salt (optional)
2 tablespoons unsalted butter, softened
2 tablespoons heavy cream
2 tablespoons lowfat milk
¼ teaspoon freshly grated nutmeg
Few grinds fresh black pepper

To prepare the pot roast, preheat the oven to 350° F.

Cook the bacon over medium heat just until limp. Drain on paper towels.

Heat the olive oil in a large Dutch oven over medium-high heat. Brown the venison, turning until all sides are brown. Drain off any excess fat. Lay the partially cooked strips of bacon on top of the meat in the Dutch oven. Add the beef broth and wine. Sprinkle with salt and pepper Tie together sprigs of fresh thyme with kitchen twine and add to the pot. Bring the broth to a boil over high heat. Cover and transfer to the oven. Bake for 1¼ hours, basting two or three times.

Add the onions, rutabaga, turnip, carrot, and garlic. Cover and bake for 1 more hour, or until meat and vegetables are tender.

Nutritional Analysis per serving (no salt added)

Calories: 643
Fat: 19.5 g
Saturated fat: 9.2 g
Cholesterol: 177 mg
High in fiber, and vitamins A and C
Sodium: 318 mg

Meanwhile, make the parsnip whipped potatoes. Put the potatoes and parsnips in a 4-quart pot and cover with water seasoned with a pinch of salt. Bring to a boil. Reduce the heat, cover, and simmer for 20 to 30 minutes or until very tender. Drain and return the parsnips and potatoes to the pot.

Mash the hot parsnips and potatoes with a potato masher or a hand-held electric mixer. Beat in the butter.

Heat the cream and milk in a small saucepan until hot but not boiling. Add to the mashed parsnips and potatoes and beat until fluffy. Season to taste with nutmeg, salt, and pepper. Set aside and keep warm.

Transfer the venison to a platter and discard the bacon. Cover and keep warm. Transfer the vegetables to a serving bowl with slotted spoon; discard the thyme.

Skim the fat from the pan juices. Boil the juices, uncovered, over high heat for 15 to 20 minutes until reduced to about 1 cup. Set aside.

Combine the softened butter and cornstarch until well blended and then add to the reduced liquid. Cook for 2 to 3 minutes, stirring, until the sauce is slightly thickened and bubbly. Cook for 2 minutes more and strain through a fine sieve. Stir in the chopped parsley and thyme.

To serve, slice the meat and arrange it with the vegetables on a serving platter. Pass the potatoes in a heated vegetable dish. Spoon sauce over the meat and vegetables or pass it separately.

Note: Venison can be mail ordered through Lucky Star Ranch, Chaumont, NY 13622, (315) 649-5519. As of press time, the venison ran about $9.25 per pound.

LARRY FORGIONE
....

Spicy Grilled Chicken with Apples and Chiles
Serves 4

This is an easy recipe that provides a nice balance of spices from the peppers and chiles and sweetness from the apples. It's also a great do-ahead recipe for stress-free cooking.

¼ cup fresh orange juice
¼ cup fresh pineapple juice
2 tablespoons fresh lemon juice
2 tablespoons fresh lime juice
1 jalapeño pepper, cored, seeded, and sliced thin
2 Anaheim peppers, cored, seeded, and sliced thin
1 small red bell pepper, cored, seeded, and sliced thin
2 tablespoons finely chopped red onion
½ teaspoon finely chopped garlic
2 tablespoons chopped parsley
¼ cup chopped fresh cilantro
4 boneless chicken breast halves, with skin
1 tablespoon vegetable oil
Salt (optional) and freshly ground black pepper
2 tart apples
2 tablespoons lightly salted butter

Combine the juices, peppers, onions, garlic, parsley, and cilantro in a bowl.

Put the chicken breasts in a shallow, nonreactive dish and pour the marinade over them. Cover and refrigerate for 4 to 6 hours, turning the chicken a few times.

Prepare a charcoal, wood, or gas grill or preheat the broiler.

Remove the chicken from the marinade and pat dry. Rub each piece with vegetable oil and season with salt and pepper. Strain the marinade, reserving the liquid and solids separately.

Grill the chicken breasts over medium heat, skin side down, for 4 to 5 minutes, until the skin is crisp and brown. Turn the breasts over and grill the other side for 3 to 4 minutes, basting from time to time with the marinade liquid.

While the chicken is grilling, peel and core the apples. Cut them into quarters and cut the quarters into slices.

Nutritional Analysis per serving (no salt added)

Calories: 297
Fat: 12.6 g
Saturated fat: 4.7 g
Cholesterol: 89 mg
Moderate source of fiber
Sodium: 84 mg
High in vitamins A, C, and E

Melt the butter in a large skillet over medium-high heat. When the butter is foaming, add the apples and stir. When the apples begin to brown, add the sliced chilis and herbs from the marinade. Stir to combine and season with salt and pepper.

Put the grilled chicken breasts in the center of a serving platter. Spoon the apple mixture around them.

Dessert

JIMMY SCHMIDT

BAKED PEAR WITH WILDFLOWER HONEY, WINE, AND VANILLA

Serves 4

Jimmy sprinkles balsamic vinegar and whole peppercorns over the pears just before serving. Although this may sound odd to the uninitiated, the vinegar is actually quite sweet and the peppercorns, which have been toasted, are crunchy bites of flavor, not sharpness. You can reduce the calorie count of this recipe by using only half the sauce. If so, each serving is only 299 calories. The other counts remain the same.

4 large, firm pears, such as Anjou or Bosc
1 cup wildflower honey or any pure honey
1 cup sweet wine, such as Riesling or sauterne
1 whole vanilla bean, split lengthwise
1 tablespoon pure vanilla extract
1 tablespoon cracked black peppercorns
¼ cup packed light brown sugar
2 tablespoons balsamic vinegar
4 sprigs mint

Preheat the oven to 400° F.

Trim the bottoms of the pears so that they stand upright and place them in an ovenproof dish large enough to hold them so that they do not touch. Mix the honey with the wine and spoon it over the pears. Add the vanilla bean. Bake the pears on the lower rack of the oven, basting very 15 minutes, for about 45 minutes, or until tender when pierced with a skewer or fork. Remove from the oven and put the pears in a shallow dish to cool.

Nutritional Analysis per serving
Calories: 447
Fat: 0.8 g
Saturated fat: 0.5 g
Cholesterol: 0 mg
Excellent source of fiber
Sodium: 11 mg

Spoon the cooking syrup and vanilla bean into a saucepan and bring to a boil over medium-high heat. Cook for 4 to 5 minutes, until the syrup thickens enough to coat the back of a spoon. Remove from the heat and strain through a fine sieve. Reserve the vanilla bean. Add the vanilla extract to the sauce.

(continued)

Put the vanilla bean on a cutting board and scrape the seeds from it with a small paring knife. Add the seeds to the sauce and discard the bean.

Toast the cracked peppercorns in a small skillet over low heat for about 3 minutes, until they smoke slightly. This minimizes the peppercorns' biting spiciness. Transfer to a plate to cool.

Using a melon ball cutter, remove the core of each pear from the base and discard. Trim the bottom of the pears again, if necessary, so that they sit flat. Set the pears in a shallow pan that fits under the broiler so that the pears will be approximately 2 inches from the heat. Sprinkle them with brown sugar and broil for about 2 minutes, until the sugar caramelizes. Rotate the pears as necessary for an even glaze.

Serve the pears with the sauce spooned over them and pooled around each. Using an eye-dropper or demitasse spoon, drizzle balsamic vinegar over the sauce. Sprinkle the peppercorns over the pears and sauce on each plate and garnish with sprigs of mint.

LARRY FORGIONE
....

OLD-FASHIONED APPLE AND CRANBERRY DUFF
Serves 4

This is an old-fashioned recipe that takes only minutes to prepare and less than thirty minutes to bake. In the eighteenth and nineteenth centuries, baked apple desserts were common in New England and elsewhere in the eastern part of the country, mostly because of the large crops of fall apples. A duff is sort of a quick variation of a cobbler and an English trifle.

Fruit
¾ cup granulated sugar
2 tablespoons quick-cooking tapioca
1 cup apple cider
1 cup cranberries
2 tablespoons applejack (apple brandy)
1 tablespoon grated fresh ginger
Zest of 1 lemon, grated
6 tart apples, such as Macoun or Northern Spy, peeled, cored, and sliced

Topping
2 large egg yolks
⅓ cup granulated sugar
1 teaspoon pure vanilla extract
2 large egg whites
¼ cup all-purpose flour
Confectioners' sugar, for dusting

To prepare the fruit, preheat the oven to 350° F and butter a 2½-quart baking dish.

Combine the sugar and tapioca in a large saucepan and stir in the apple cider. Cook over medium heat, stirring, until the sugar dissolves. Stir in the cranberries, applejack, ginger, lemon zest, and apples. Raise the heat to high and bring to a boil. Lower the heat to a simmer, cover, and cook for about 4 minutes, until the apples are slightly softened. Spoon the fruit into the baking dish.

To prepare the topping, beat the egg yolks and sugar with an electric mixer for 3 to 4 minutes, until thick and lemon colored. Stir in the vanilla.

> *Nutritional Analysis*
> *per serving*
>
> *Calories: 480*
> *Fat: 5.3 g*
> *Saturated fat: 2.1 g*
> *Cholesterol: 111 mg*
> *Good source of fiber*
> *Sodium: 35 mg*

In another bowl and using clean beaters, beat the egg whites with an electric mixer until soft peaks form. Fold the flour into the whites. Fold the whites into the egg yolk and sugar mixture.

Pour the topping over the fruit, spreading it gently with a rubber spatula to cover the surface. Bake, uncovered, for 20 to 25 minutes until the topping is golden brown and begins to pull away from the sides of the pan. Let the duff cool slightly. Sprinkle with confectioners' sugar and serve warm.

ALICE WATERS
....

BAKED FIGS IN RED WINE

Serves 4

In keeping with Alice's philosophy of eating the best of any given season, here is a simple and wonderful way to take advantage of early autumn's crop of rich, juicy figs. As with Jimmy's pears, on page 151, this dessert uses a little pepper to bring out its flavor. It's important, too, to use good wine.

16 ripe figs
⅓ cup sweet red dessert wine or port, or a combination of the two
Few grinds fresh black pepper
3 to 4 sprigs fresh thyme

Preheat the oven to 375° F.

> *Nutritional Analysis*
> *per serving*
>
> *Calories: 168*
> *Fat: < 1 g*
> *Saturated fat: < 1 g*
> *Cholesterol: 0 mg*
> *High source of fiber*
> *Sodium: 3 mg*

Cut the stems from the tops of the figs and the tiny leaves from the bottoms, taking care not to cut into the flesh any more than necessary. Slice the figs in half lengthwise.

Arrange the fig halves, skin side up, in a single layer in a ceramic or glass baking dish. Pour the wine over the figs and season with pepper to taste. Scatter the thyme over the figs.

Bake, uncovered, for about 35 minutes, until the figs are soft and browned and the wine reduces to a syrup. Discard the thyme. Serve the figs slightly warm.

WINTER
RECIPES

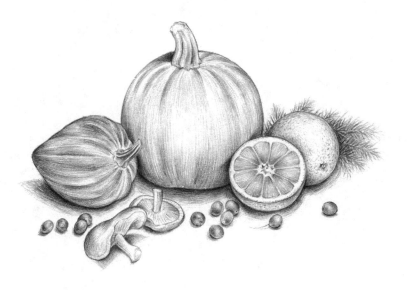

Breakfast

ALICE WATERS
....

BANANA PANCAKES
Serves 4

Alice makes these sweet wintertime pancakes with a whole wheat batter lightened by egg whites and flavored by sliced ripe bananas. Straining the batter before mixing it with the whipped egg whites removes lumps. Serve the pancakes with a little sugar-free jam or maple syrup—about a tablespoon per serving should provide good flavor without adding excessive calories (see below).

½ cup whole wheat pastry flour
½ cup unbleached all-purpose flour
1 teaspoon baking powder
Scant pinch kosher salt
1 egg yolk
½ cup buttermilk
½ cup low-fat milk
1 teaspoon safflower oil
1½ large bananas, peeled and sliced very thin
3 egg whites

In a large bowl, mix both flours and the baking powder with the salt. Whisk to combine thoroughly and make a well in the center of the dry ingredients.

In another bowl, whisk the egg yolk, buttermilk, low-fat milk, and oil together. Pour the wet ingredients into the well in the dry ingredients and whisk thoroughly without overmixing. Strain the batter through a fine sieve into another bowl. Gently stir the sliced bananas into the batter.

Beat the egg whites to soft peaks. Fold gently into the batter, mixing thoroughly but taking care not to deflate the batter.

Heat an iron skillet over medium-low hat. When it is hot, put a few drops of oil in the pan and tilt it so that the oil covers the surface. Using a small ladle, spoon a tablespoon or two of batter for each pancake into the pan. There should be enough batter to make 16 pancakes. Cook the pancakes for about 1½ minutes on each side until nicely browned. Serve hot with maple syrup or jam.

Nutritional Analysis per serving

Calories: 252
Fat: 8.4 g
Saturated fat: 1.6 g
Cholesterol: 56 mg
Moderate source of fiber
Sodium: 30 mg

With 1 tablespoon topping, add:
Sugar-free jam: 30 calories per serving
Maple syrup: 50 calories per serving
"Light" maple syrup: 30 calories per serving
Confectioners' sugar: 30 calories per serving

JIMMY SCHMIDT
....

PEAR, PARSNIP, AND POTATO PANCAKES
Serves 4

A giant-sized pancake that you cut into four pieces for serving makes a great weekend break-fast or brunch dish. Jimmy's calls for potatoes and parsnips as well as pears for a substantial meal that supplies lots of good fiber and terrific flavor.

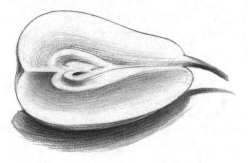

1 baking potato, peeled
2 large parsnips, peeled
1 cup all-purpose flour
½ cup granulated sugar
1 teaspoon baking powder
1 large egg, beaten
¼ cup low-fat milk
Kosher salt (optional)
Few grinds fresh black pepper
2 tablespoons unsalted butter
4 large pears, such as Comice, Bosc, or Anjou,
    peeled, cored, sliced, and rubbed with lemon
Confectioner's sugar
4 sprigs mint

Preheat the oven to 375° F.

Grate the potato and parsnips in a food processor fitted with the fine grating blade. Transfer to a colander and rinse under cold run-ning water for about 3 minutes until the water runs clear to re-move excess starch. Drain well.

Nutritional Analysis per serving (no salt added)

Calories: 502
Fat: 8.4 g
Saturated fat: 4.1 g
Cholesterol: 63 mg
High in fiber
Sodium: 138 mg

Meanwhile, bring a large pot of water to a boil. Add the grated po-tato and parsnips and cook for no longer than 1 to 2 minutes over high heat, until the vegetables are blanched and slightly firm to the bite. Drain well and transfer to a large bowl.

In another bowl, combine the flour, ¼ cup of the granulated sugar, and the baking powder. Add this to the grated vegetables and toss to coat evenly. Mix together the egg and milk and add slowly, stirring, until the batter is smooth and thick. Season to taste with salt and pepper.

Melt the butter in a large nonstick, ovenproof skillet over medium-high heat. Add the pears and remaining ¼ cup of sugar and cook for about 2 minutes, until softened. Spread the pears evenly across the bottom of the skillet. Pour the batter over the pears, tilting the skil-let slightly so that the batter fills all the spaces around and between the fruit. Transfer the skillet to the oven for 6 to 8 minutes, until the pancake is golden and slightly resilient to the touch.

Remove the skillet from the oven and invert a plate over the pancake. With one hand on the plate, quickly turn the pan and plate over in one motion to release the pancake onto the plate. Sprinkle confectioners' sugar over the top. Garnish with mint and serve by cutting the pancake into four equal pieces.

LARRY FORGIONE

SWEET CORN PORRIDGE WITH DRIED FRUITS
Serves 4

Cornmeal, cooked in scalded milk and sweetened with brown sugar and maple syrup, cooks into a porridge similar to corn pudding. The dried fruit may be easier to chop if you toss it with a little flour first. You can buy an assortment of fruits, often already chopped, or mix and match your own.

3 cups 1% low-fat milk
2 tablespoons brown sugar
1 tablespoon maple syrup
Scant ⅓ cup stone-ground cornmeal
1 cup assorted diced dried fruit, such as apricots, apples, raisins, currants, and prunes
Kosher salt (optional)
Few grinds fresh black pepper
1 tablespoon unsalted butter

Put the milk, brown sugar, and syrup in a saucepan and cook over high heat until scalded (small bubbles begin to form around the edges but milk does not quite boil). Lower the heat to a simmer and slowly add the cornmeal, stirring continually, for 3 to 4 minutes, until the milk and cornmeal are the consistency of mush (similar to grits and Cream of Wheat). Stir in the dried fruit.

Season with a pinch of salt and pepper and stir in the butter. Spoon into bowls and serve with more brown sugar, syrup, and butter, if desired.

Nutritional Analysis per serving (no salt added)

Calories: 250
Fat: 5.4 g
Saturated fat: 3.1 g
Cholesterol: 15 mg
Moderate source of fiber and good source of vitamin A
Sodium: 103 mg

Lunch and Salads

JIMMY SCHMIDT
....

ROASTED BEETS, ENDIVE, AND FRISÉE SALAD

Serves 4

Beets are one of the better vegetables to buy fresh in the winter. If possible, buy them with healthy-looking greens attached and trim them so that an inch or so of the greens stays on the root during cooking. Never peel beets before cooking them—you will lose valuable nutrients and color. They are also far easier to peel after cooking—the skins slip off. In this recipe, Jimmy roasts the beets for rich, sweet flavor.

4 large beets (about 1 pound)
2 tablespoons red wine vinegar
2 tablespoons prepared horseradish
¼ cup nonfat yogurt
2 tablespoons extra-virgin olive oil
Kosher salt (optional)
Few grinds fresh black pepper
2 Belgian endives
1 large head or 3 tiny heads baby frisée (curly endive), torn into bite-size pieces

Preheat the oven to 375° F.

Put the whole beets with their skins on in an ovenproof pan. Bake on the lower rack of the oven for about 45 minutes, until tender when pierced with a fork. Remove from the oven, place on a wire rack, and cool to room temperature. When cool, peel with a paring knife and cut into ¼-inch slices. Cut the slices into ¼-inch julienne and transfer to a small bowl.

In another small bowl, whisk together the vinegar, horseradish, yogurt, and olive oil. Season the dressing to taste with salt and pepper.

Nutritional Analysis per serving (without added salt)

Calories: 136
Fat: 7.2 g
Saturated fat: 1 g
Cholesterol: 0.3 mg
Moderate source of fiber and good source of vitamin A
Sodium: 127 mg

Peel 16 of the large outer leaves from the 2 endives. On each of 4 individual plates, arrange 4 of the leaves at the 4 compass points.

Cut the remaining endive crosswise into ¼-inch slices. Transfer to a medium bowl. Add the frisée and about three-quarters of the dressing. Toss to combine. Spoon some salad into the center of each plate, with the endive leaves peeking out from under it.

Add the remaining dressing to the beets and toss to coat. Divide the beets among the 4 plates over the frisée and endive. Season with black pepper and serve.

JIMMY SCHMIDT
....

CALAMARI, WHITE BEAN, AND RED LENTIL RAGOUT

Serves 4

Calamari, or squid, is a popular ingredient in Mediterannean countries and slowly but surely is gaining acceptance here. And for good reason! Ask the fishmonger to prepare the calamari for you, or buy it whole and cut it up yourself. The beans for this ragout need to soak over- night—so plan ahead. Although lentils are normally not presoaked, this recipe requires it.

4 ounces dried white beans, picked over
2 ounces dried red lentils, picked over
1 onion, peeled and quartered
2 bay leaves
2 teaspoons fresh thyme leaves
1 tablespoon whole black peppercorns
1 bunch Italian flat-leaf parsley, leaves chopped (reserve 4 sprigs for garnish)
    and stems reserved
2 tablespoons extra-virgin olive oil
2 cloves garlic, peeled and minced
1 cup dry white wine
2 cups homemade vegetable broth (page 194) or low-sodium vegetable
    broth from bouillon cubes
Kosher salt (optional)
Freshly ground black pepper
1 pound small calamari, cleaned, body cut into rounds, and tentacles
    quartered lengthwise

Put the white beans in a bowl and cover with enough water to cover them by 2 inches. Put the red lentils in a separate bowl and cover with water the same way. Refrigerate both for 8 hours or overnight. (Or use the quick-soaking method; see Note below.) Drain the white beans in a colander and discard the soaking water. Repeat with the lentils. (Keep the beans and lentils separate.) Rinse both well under running water. Set aside the lentils.

To prepare the ragout, put the white beans and the onion into a me- dium saucepan and add enough fresh water to cover by 2 inches. Tie the bay leaves, half the thyme, the peppercorns, and parsley stems in cheesecloth and add to the beans. Bring to a simmer and cook over medium heat for about 1 hour and 45 minutes, until tender. Remove from the heat, discard the spice sack and onion, and drain the beans in a colander.

Heat the olive oil in a large nonstick skillet over medium-high heat. Add the garlic and cook for about 2 minutes, until golden brown. Add the remaining thyme and cook for about 2 minutes, until wilted. Add the white wine and 2 cups of vegetable broth and bring to a boil. Add the lentils and cook for about 5 minutes, until softened but still firm to the

*Nutritional Analysis
per serving (without
added salt)*

Calories: 339
Fat: 9.5 g
Saturated fat: 1.6 g
Cholesterol: 247 mg
High source of fiber
Sodium: 338 mg

(continued)

bite. Add the white beans and cook for about 10 minutes, until the liquids are reduced to a sauce that lightly coats the beans. Season to taste with salt and a generous amount of black pepper.

Add the calamari and chopped parsley and cook for about 1 minute, until the calamari is opaque; do not overcook.

Spoon the ragout into 4 rimmed soup plates. Season with black pepper to taste and garnish each serving with a sprig of parsley. Serve.

Note: To use the quick-soaking method, put the beans and lentils into separate large pots and add enough water to cover by 2 to 3 inches. Bring to a boil, reduce the heat, and simmer for 2 minutes. Remove from the heat and soak for 1 hour. Drain and discard the soaking water. Rinse well. This eliminates the 8 hours of soaking.

JIMMY SCHMIDT

VEGETABLE BLACK BEAN CHILI
Serves 8

Jimmy's black bean chili is chock-full of wintertime vegetables—squash, fennel, and parsnip. The beans are a good source of fiber and nutrients, and with only a little forethought are very easy to prepare. Make this chili as fiery as you like by selecting the hot pepper you like best. Jimmy suggests a dried pasilla, which is a long, tapered purple-black chile with a rich smoky intensity that is not too overpowering in the heat department. Or you may leave out the hot pepper altogether.

½ pound dried black turtle beans
4 cloves garlic, unpeeled
¼ cup plus 2 teaspoons extra-virgin olive oil
2 cups diced onion
1 tablespoon chili powder
1 large dried pasilla chile or another hot pepper (optional)
1 tablespoon salt
Few grinds fresh black pepper
¼ cup fresh lime juice
2 cups diced winter squash such as buttercup, butternut, or acorn
1 bulb fennel, trimmed and diced
1 parsnip, peeled and diced
½ cup low-fat yogurt
½ cup snipped fresh scallion greens

Put the black beans in a large pot and add enough water to cover by 2 to 3 inches. Refrigerate for 8 hours or overnight. Drain the beans in a colander, discarding the soaking water, and rinse well under running water. (Or use the quick-soaking method; see Note below.)

Preheat the oven to 400° F.

In an ovenproof dish, coat the garlic cloves with the 2 teaspoons of oil. Set the dish on the lower rack of the oven and bake for about 30 minutes, until the garlic skin is brown and the inside flesh is tender. Remove from the oven and allow to cool to room temperature. Peel to expose the tender inner vegetable or squeeze by hand to force the garlic from the skin. Mince the garlic.

Pour the ¼ cup of olive oil into a large pot, add the onion, and sauté over high heat for about 3 minutes, until the onions are tender. Add the chili powder and cook for 1 minute. Add the drained beans and pasilla or hot chile pepper. Add cold water until the water level is 1 inch above the beans. Add half the salt and season to taste with black pepper.

Bring to a simmer, reduce the heat to medium, and cook for about 1½ to 2 hours, until the beans are tender. Remove the pasilla or hot pepper. Stir in the minced roasted garlic and the lime juice. Season with salt and pepper to taste.

Add the squash, fennel, and parsnip and cook for about 7 minutes, until the vegetables are tender. Ladle the chili into 4 warm bowls. Top with yogurt and scallion greens and serve immediately.

Note: To use the quick-soaking method, put the beans into a large pot and add enough water to cover by 2 to 3 inches. Bring to a boil, reduce the heat, and simmer for 2 minutes. Remove from the heat and soak for 1 hour. Drain and discard the soaking water. Rinse well. This eliminates the 8 hours of soaking.

Nutritional Analysis per serving

Calories: 212
Cholesterol: 93 mg
Fat: 7.6 g
Saturated fat: 1.2 g
Excellent source of fiber and vitamin A
Sodium: 842 mg

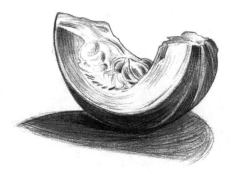

ALICE WATERS
....

SMOKED FISH AND CELERY ROOT SALAD
Serves 4

What a wonderful idea! Smoked fish, which is easy to buy at the local deli or specialty counter in the grocery, over a light, refreshing salad made with celery root. Make sure the fish is of the best quality.

¼ cup extra-virgin olive oil
2 teaspoons fresh lemon juice
2 teaspoons Champagne vinegar
Kosher salt (optional)
Few grinds fresh black pepper
⅓ small celery root, trimmed (2 to 3 ounces)
½ pound smoked trout, salmon, tuna, sable (black cod), or sturgeon, boned if necessary
About 6 ounces frisée (curly endive) or Belgian endive
1 scant cup fresh chervil leaves
¼ teaspoon grated lemon zest

Whisk the olive oil, lemon juice, and vinegar until emulsified. Season the dressing to taste with salt and pepper. Set aside.

Cut the celery root into matchsticks that are about ¹⁄₁₆ inch wide. Put them in a small bowl and add fresh water to cover. Add salt until the water tastes like sea water. Let stand for about 15 minutes, until wilted. Drain the celery root, rinse in fresh water, and set aside.

Break the fish into 1-inch pieces. Check carefully for stray bones.

Put the frisée, chervil leaves, celery root, and lemon zest into a bowl and sprinkle with a little salt and pepper. Pour about three-quarters of the dressing over the salad and toss gently but thoroughly. Put the salad in the center of a serving platter and top with the smoked fish. Drizzle the remaining dressing over the fish and serve immediately.

Nutritional Analysis per serving (without added salt)

Calories: 261
Fat: 21.1 g
Saturated fat: 3.8 g
Cholesterol: 54 mg
Relatively low source of fiber
High in vitamin A
Good source of vitamin E
Sodium: 195 mg

ALICE WATERS

WINTER VEGETABLE SALADS
Serves 4

Alice relies on wilted winter greens as the foundation for this medley of salads made with classic winter vegetables: beets, celery root, and carrots. Note the relatively high fat count in this recipe—but also note that very little of it is saturated fat.

Salads
3 beets (about 8 ounces in all)
1 small celery root (about 8 ounces)
Kosher salt (optional)
3 large carrots (about 8 ounces in all)
1 teaspoon extra-virgin olive oil
Few grinds fresh black pepper
About 4 ounces greens, such as frisée (curly endive), dandelion, rocket, or chard
2 tablespoons finely chopped parsley

Vinaigrette
1 shallot, chopped fine
1½ teaspoons Champagne or white wine vinegar
¼ cup extra-virgin olive oil
Kosher salt (optional)
Few grinds fresh black pepper

Preheat the oven to 350° F.

Scrub the beets gently and lay them in a shallow roasting pan. Sprinkle 3 tablespoons of water over them and roast for about 1 hour, until fork tender. Let them cool, trim away the stems, and peel the beets. Cut them into ¹⁄₁₆-inch-thick slices and then cut the slices into matchsticks. Set aside.

Cut the stem and root end from the celery root and then peel and halve it. Cut the halves into ¹⁄₁₆-inch-thick slices and then cut the slices into matchsticks. Put the matchsticks in a small bowl and add enough fresh water to cover. Add salt until the water tastes like sea water. Let stand for about 15 minutes, until wilted. Drain the celery root, rinse in fresh water, and set aside.

Peel the carrots and cut into 3-inch pieces. Slice the pieces lengthwise into 1/16-inch-thick slices and then cut the slices into matchsticks. Put 2 cups of water into a saucepan and add salt until it tastes like sea water. Bring to a gentle boil and cook the carrot matchsticks for about 4 minutes. Drain, rinse in fresh water for about 30 seconds, and set aside to cool.

(continued)

Nutritional Analysis per serving (no salt added)

Calories: 197
Fat: 15 g
Saturated fat: 2 g
Cholesterol: 0 mg
Good source of fiber and vitamin E
Very high in vitamin A
Sodium: 173 mg

In a skillet over medium-high heat combine 1 tablespoon of water, the oil, and salt and pepper to taste. Add the greens and cook, tossing, for about 2 minutes, until tender and wilted. Lift the greens from the pan with tongs and transfer to a small bowl to cool.

To make the vinaigrette, mix the chopped shallot with the vinegar in a ceramic or glass bowl. Let sit for 30 minutes. Whisk the oil into the vinegar until emulsified and season to taste with salt and pepper.

Toss the beets, celery root, carrots, and greens individually with a little dressing. Toss the celery root and carrots with a tablespoon of parsley each. Mound the salads on a cool platter and serve.

Alice Waters

Pasta with Mushrooms, Fennel, and Thyme

Serves 4

Dried mushrooms are wonderful to have on hand to provide earthy flavor in all sorts of dishes. They rehydrate in about thirty minutes and then can be used as though they were fresh. Although Alice's first choice is morels for this recipe, you can use other dried mushrooms. Dried cepes are also called porcini.

1½ ounces dried morels, cepes, or chanterelles
2 cups hot water
½ fennel bulb, trimmed and halved again
1 carrot, peeled
1 onion, peeled
2 tablespoons extra-virgin olive oil
1 clove garlic, peeled and minced
1 teaspoon minced fresh thyme leaves
Fresh lemon juice
1 teaspoon kosher salt
Few grinds fresh black pepper
12 ounces dried linguine
3 tablespoons finely chopped parsley

Soak the morels in the hot water, covered, for about 30 minutes. Drain and reserve the mushroom liquor. Strain the liquor through a fine sieve or a double layer of cheesecloth into a small bowl. Cut the mushrooms in half lengthwise or in quarters, depending on their size, and set aside.

Cut the fennel bulb halves, carrot, and onion into 1/16-inch dice. Heat the olive oil and 1 tablespoon of water in a large saucepan over medium heat and cook the vegetables and garlic, covered, for about 15 minutes, until soft and sweet. Add the mushrooms, ¼ cup of mushroom liquor, ¼ cup of water, and the thyme. Cook for another 5 minutes and season to taste with a squeeze of lemon juice and salt and pepper. Set aside and keep warm.

Bring 6 quarts of salted water to a boil in a large pot and cook the pasta for 10 to 12 minutes, until firm and resilient. Drain the pasta and add it to the pan holding the mushroom mixture. Add the parsley and toss well. Transfer to a warm bowl and serve immediately.

Nutritional Analysis per serving

Calories: 436
Fat: 8.4 g
Saturated fat: 1.16 g
Cholesterol: 0 mg
Good source of fiber and vitamin A
Sodium: 484 mg

LARRY FORGIONE

WINTER PEAR, ENDIVE, AND FRISÉE SALAD WITH CRUMBLED BLUE CHEESE AND RED WINE VINAIGRETTE
Serves 4

A little bit of blue cheese goes a long way toward making a salad taste special and adds its own warm depth of flavor that stands up to a robust red wine vinaigrette. But, to reduce calories and fat, leave it out of the salad if you prefer. Larry uses small Seckel pears for this winter salad—a variety of American pear that is dark green with a red cheek and is in season from early fall through midwinter. Western Seckel pears are a little larger than Eastern varieties, and have a sweeter flavor, too. Other types of pears may also be used.

1 tablespoon red wine vinegar
½ teaspoon balsamic vinegar
½ teaspoon red wine
1 tablespoon extra-virgin olive oil
⅛ teaspoon minced garlic
1 tablespoon finely chopped shallot or white part of scallion
1 teaspoon chopped fresh rosemary or thyme
Kosher salt (optional)
Few grinds fresh black pepper
1 head Belgian endive
2 heads frisée (curly endive)
4 Seckel pears or other firm small pears
1 ounce blue cheese

In a small bowl, whisk together the vinegars, red wine, and olive oil. Add the garlic, shallot, and rosemary and whisk to blend. Season to taste with salt and pepper. Set the dressing aside.

Nutritional Analysis per serving (no salt added)

Calories: 176
Fat: 6.4 g
Saturated fat: 1.9 g
Cholesterol: 5 mg
High in fiber and vitamin A
Sodium: 114 mg

(continued)

Trim the bottoms of the endive and frisée and separate the leaves into a bowl. Cut the pears in half and cut out the cores. Cut each half into 4 pieces and add to the bowl. Add 2 tablespoons of the vinaigrette to the salad and toss.

Arrange the salad on four plates and crumble the blue cheese over each one. Drizzle the remaining dressing over the salads and serve.

LARRY FORGIONE

WARM CHICKEN SALAD WITH WALNUT SHERRY VINAIGRETTE

Serves 4

Warm salads are a pleasure in the wintertime, because while they are refreshingly light, they are not the cool, crisp customers of summer. The walnut oil rounds out the flavor of this salad and gives the chicken a slight nuttiness.

4 (4-ounce) boneless, skinless chicken breast halves
Kosher salt (optional)
Few grinds fresh black pepper
1 tablespoon walnut or extra-virgin olive oil
⅓ cup chopped walnuts
2 scallions, sliced fine
¼ teaspoon minced garlic
3 tablespoons cream sherry
3 tablespoons white wine vinegar
2 tablespoons extra-virgin olive oil
6 to 8 cups assorted lettuces such as arugula, red leaf, and oak leaf lettuce,
    and watercress, washed and patted dry
2 tablespoons finely chopped chives

Cut each chicken breast crosswise into 6 to 8 strips. Season with salt and pepper. Heat the walnut oil in a large, nonstick skillet over medium-high heat. Add the chicken strips in batches, being careful not to overcrowd the pan, and cook for 2 to 3 minutes on each side until cooked through and lightly browned. Remove the cooked chicken strips to a plate. Continue until all the chicken is cooked.

Add the chopped walnuts to the pan and cook for 1 to 2 minutes. Add the scallions and garlic and stir briefly. Add the sherry and let it boil for 1 minute. Add the vinegar and olive oil.

When the vinegar and olive oil are heated, return the cooked chicken to the pan and toss briefly.

Nutritional Analysis per serving (no salt added)

Calories: 317
Fat: 19.2
Saturated fat: 2.6 g
Cholesterol: 72 mg
Moderate source of vitamins A and E and fiber
Sodium: 71 mg

Toss the lettuces with 1 tablespoon of the dressing from the skillet. Divide the lettuces among 4 serving plates. Put some chicken strips on each plate and spoon some dressing over the top. Sprinkle with the chives and additional freshly ground black pepper before serving.

LARRY FORGIONE

SEARED SEA SCALLOPS WITH CRANBERRIES AND HICKORY NUTS

Serves 4

Sweet sea scallops, briefly sautéed and then set atop a lightly dressed salad of bitter greens, are offset by a chunky sauce made from tart cranberries, scallions, and buttery hickory nuts.

2 tablespoons extra-virgin olive oil
1 tablespoon red wine vinegar
1 teaspoon finely chopped shallot or white part of scallion plus 1 tablespoon
    thinly sliced shallot
Kosher salt (optional)
Few grinds fresh black pepper
3 cups torn assorted greens, such as arugula, red leaf lettuce, and oak leaf
    lettuce, washed and patted dry
12 jumbo sea scallops
1 teaspoon butter
¼ cup coarsely chopped hickory nuts or pecans
½ cup fresh cranberries, halved or coarsely chopped
½ teaspoon finely chopped fresh rosemary
2 tablespoons cream sherry

Whisk all but 1 teaspoon of the olive oil with the vinegar in a small bowl. Add the shallot and whisk again. Season the vinaigrette to taste with salt and pepper.

In a bowl, toss the greens together. Spoon the vinaigrette over the greens and toss. Divide evenly among 4 plates.

Season the scallops with salt and pepper. In a large, nonstick skillet, heat the remaining teaspoon of olive oil over medium-high heat until hot. Add the scallops and cook for about 2 minutes on each side, until they are just pink in the center. Remove and keep warm.

(continued)

Nutritional Analysis per serving (no salt added)

Calories: 204
Fat: 14.7 g
Saturated fat: 2.2 g
Cholesterol: 21 mg
Relatively low source of fiber
Good source of vitamins A and E
Sodium: 126 mg

Reduce the heat to medium low. Add the butter to the skillet and, when it melts, add the nuts. Cook for 1 minute, stirring. Add the cranberries, sliced shallot, rosemary, and sherry. Cook for 1 minute or until the sauce is thickened and the cranberries are soft.

To serve, arrange 3 scallops on top of each plate of greens. Spoon the cranberry–nut mixture around each salad and serve immediately.

Appetizers

ALICE WATERS
. . . .
FISH TARTARE WITH CAPERS, LEMON, AND SHALLOTS
Serves 4

Because the fish has an opportunity to marinate in a dressing made with lemon juice, it is not absolutely raw when you eat it—only light, flavorful, and wonderful. The acid in the juice breaks down fibers in the fish and "cooks" it in a manner similar to seviche. Buy fresh fish from a reliable market and use one kind or a combination of all three. Serve this on endive leaves or small toasts.

12 ounces fresh tuna, halibut, or salmon
1½ teaspoons capers, drained, rinsed, and chopped
1 tablespoon finely chopped shallot
2 teaspoons extra-virgin olive oil
Juice of ½ lemon
2 teaspoons finely chopped chervil
½ teaspoon kosher salt
Few grinds fresh black pepper

Check the fish for bones and cut away any dark fat from the fish with a very sharp knife. Cut the fish into thin strips about ⅛ inch across. Cut the strips into fine dice.

Using a large, sharp knife, mince the fish until it is smooth and even but not a paste. Transfer the fish to a bowl and add the capers, shallot, olive oil, lemon juice, and chervil. Season to taste with salt and pepper. Cover and refrigerate for 1 hour before serving.

Nutritional Analysis per serving

Calories: 117
Fat: 4.2 g
Saturated fat: 0.6 g
Cholesterol: 27 mg
Relatively low source of fiber
Sodium: 275 mg

LARRY FORGIONE
······················

STEAMED MUSSELS WITH FENNEL IN AN ORANGE BROTH
Serves 4

Mussels are abundant among available mollusks in our fish markets. They are harvested on both the East and West coasts, sold in their familiar deep blue shells. But often they are passed over for other seafood, which is a shame since they are tender and delicious and an excellent source of protein. And like all mollusks, they are very low in fat. In this recipe, Larry prepares them with fennel and orange—two distinct flavors that complement the mussels' mildness. This is a delightful first course and would also make a good light meal.

Mussels are sold by the quart, the dozen, or the pound, and for this recipe you will need about two quarts (three pounds or four dozen), which should give you enough mussels even if you have to discard a few. As well as discarding any that don't open during cooking, check them before cooking and toss out any that are overloaded with dark mud. You can determine this by pressing the shell. The beard referred to in the recipe is a tuft of fibers that protrudes from the shell. These are what the mussel uses to anchor itself to rocks. It easily scrubs off or pulls off with pliers or strong tweezers. Mussels are at their best in late winter through early spring, as well as late summer.

1 small fennel bulb
4 dozen unshucked mussels
1 cup dry white wine
1 cup dry vermouth
1 cup homemade chicken broth (page 193) or low-sodium canned broth
2 teaspoons minced garlic
1 bay leaf
¼ cup heavy cream
Zest of 1 orange, blanched in boiling water for 1 minute and diced fine
2 tablespoons finely chopped fresh basil
1 tablespoon finely chopped parsley

Trim the fennel bulb and separate the outer branches from the center (or heart). Roughly chop the outer branches. Cut the center in half. Remove the core and slice the bulb very thin.

Wash the mussels under cold running water and scrub with a coarse brush to remove any dirt. Do not submerge the mussels in fresh water. Press lightly on any open mussels and discard any that do not close up. Remove the beards by scrubbing or pulling gently with your fingers or a clean needle-nose pliers.

Put the mussels, white wine, vermouth, chicken broth, garlic, and bay leaf in a large saucepan. Cover and bring to a boil over high heat. Lower the heat and simmer for 4 to 5 minutes, until the mussels open. Remove the mussels with a slotted spoon, discarding any that have not opened. Put the mussels in a deep bowl and cover with a damp cloth to keep warm.

*Nutritional Analysis
per serving*

*Calories: 255
Fat: 9.4 g
Saturated fat: 4.2 g
Cholesterol: 62 mg
Moderate source of
fiber and high in vita-
min A
Sodium: 672 mg*

(continued)

Increase the heat to high. Let the liquid boil for 6 to 8 minutes, until reduced by half. Add the cream, return to a boil, and simmer for 3 to 4 minutes. Strain through a fine sieve or cheesecloth into a second saucepan.

Add the blanched orange zest, basil, and parsley to the second saucepan. Continue to simmer for 1 to 2 minutes more.

Meanwhile, remove the top shells from the mussels and discard. Divide the mussels on their half-shells among 4 shallow soup bowls. Spoon the hot broth over the mussels and serve immediately.

JIMMY SCHMIDT
....

GRILLED ENDIVE WITH PARSLEY AND GREEN PEPPERCORNS
Serves 4

Jimmy grills endive leaves for this light first course with a burst of strong flavors. You can broil the endive, but, as with grilling, take great care that they do not overcook. Green peppercorns are sold in brine in most groceries and specialty shops.

4 Belgian endives, trimmed and quartered lengthwise
3 tablespoons extra-virgin olive oil
2 cloves garlic, peeled and minced
Kosher salt (optional)
Few grinds fresh black pepper
¼ cup balsamic vinegar
1 tablespoon rinsed and finely chopped green peppercorns
¼ cup chopped parsley
4 shaved slices Parmesan cheese (optional)

Combine the endive, olive oil, and garlic in a bowl. Season lightly with salt and pepper. Mix well and allow to marinate for at least 30 minutes.

Prepare a charcoal, wood, or gas grill or perheat the broiler.

Lift the endive from the marinade and lay it on the grill or under the broiler. Cook for about 3 minutes, until fork tender. Turn over and cook for about 1 minute longer, until hot all the way through. Divide the endive among 4 serving plates, arranging the grilled quarters in a fan shape.

Combine the vinegar and green peppercorns in a small bowl. Spoon over the endive. Sprinkle with parsley and black pepper. Top with shaved Parmesan cheese, if desired.

Nutritional Analysis per serving (no added salt; ½ ounce cheese per serving)

Calories: 167
Fat: 11.2 g
Saturated fat: 3.5 g
Cholesterol: 10.2 mg
Sodium: 298 mg
Excellent source of vitamin A
Moderate in fiber and good source of vitamin E

Dinner

LARRY FORGIONE
. . . .

HONEY-GLAZED GROUPER
Serves 4

As it broils, grouper, a North Atlantic swimmer, stands up to basting with a sweet-tart mixture of honey and mustard. Larry serves it with a vinegar-based red onion sauce for a tempting combination of flavors and textures. Grouper is usually readily available, but you can substitute sea bass, striped bass, tilefish, or red snapper.

1 tablespoon plus 1½ teaspoons olive oil
3 large red onions, peeled, halved, and sliced
4 shallots, peeled and sliced
Kosher salt (optional)
Few grinds fresh black pepper
¾ cup red wine
¼ cup red wine vinegar
2 tablespoons unsalted butter, at room temperature
4 (6-ounce) grouper fillets
2 tablespoons honey
1 teaspoon dry mustard
¼ teaspoon minced garlic
2 tablespoons minced fresh chives

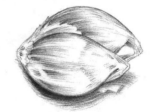

Preheat the broiler and position the broiling rack on the center rung.

Heat 1 tablespoon of oil in a large nonstick skillet over high heat. Add the sliced onions and shallots and cook for 6 to 8 minutes, stirring occasionally, until the onions brown. Season with salt and pepper and add the red wine and vinegar. Cook for 6 to 8 minutes longer, until almost all the wine evaporates. Remove the pan from the heat and stir in the butter. Season again with salt and pepper and set aside to keep warm.

Meanwhile, brush the remaining 1½ teaspoons of olive oil on the broiler tray. Season the grouper with salt and pepper and place the fish, rounded side up, on the tray.

Combine the honey, mustard, and garlic. Brush about half this mixture on the fish and broil for 2 to 3 minutes. Brush the remaining honey on the fish and raise the pan up to rung so that it is close to the heat. Cook for 2 to 3 minutes longer.

Spoon some of the glazed onions on the center of each of 4 plates and top with a grouper fillet. Sprinkle with chives and serve.

Nutritional Analysis per serving (no salt added)

Calories: 338
Fat: 13.2 g
Saturated fat: 4.7 g
Cholesterol: 76 mg
Relatively low source of fiber
High in vitamin A
Sodium: 76 mg

LARRY FORGIONE
....

SEARED FILLETS OF PORK WITH CHILI SPICES AND MAPLE-WHIPPED SWEET POTATOES

Serves 4

Pork is available all year long but we tend to associate it with fall and winter cooking—perhaps because in the days when America was an agrarian country, hogs were butchered late in the fall. Although most of the meat was cured and smoked, fresh pork was happily eaten during the ensuing weeks. Sweet potatoes also are considered a cold weather food and team perfectly with pork. They are also one of the best natural sources of beta carotene (vitamin A). This recipe calls for slices from a center-cut loin of pork; they are also called escallops or medallions.

8 (3-ounce) center-cut pork loin fillets, completely trimmed of any fat
2 tablespoons chili powder
2 teaspoons cumin
1 teaspoon kosher salt
1 teaspoon freshly ground black pepper
4 sweet potatoes
1 tablespoon low-fat sour cream, at room temperature
2 tablespoons pure maple syrup
1 teaspoon extra-virgin olive oil
1 onion, peeled and sliced
1 red bell pepper, halved, seeded, and cut into strips
1 poblano pepper, halved, seeded, and cut into strips
1 cup homemade chicken broth (page 193) or low-sodium canned broth
1 tablespoon unsalted butter, at room temperature

Preheat the oven to 375° F.

With a mallet, gently pound the pork fillets until they are about ½ inch thick. Combine the chili powder, cumin, salt, and pepper. Generously season the pork on both sides with half the seasoning mixture. Cover with plastic wrap and refrigerate until needed.

Bake the sweet potatoes for 40 to 45 minutes, until tender. Remove and let cool until cool enough to handle. Cut each potato in half and scoop the flesh into a bowl. Add the sour cream and maple syrup. Mash the potatoes with a potato masher or whisk until smooth. Season with salt and pepper. Spoon into a covered casserole dish and keep warm.

In a large nonstick skillet, heat the olive oil. Sear the pork over high heat for 1 to 2 minutes on each side. Transfer to a platter and set aside to keep warm.

Nutritional Analysis per serving

Calories: 533
Fat: 22.9 g
Saturated fat: 8.4 g
Cholesterol: 125 mg
Good source of fiber
Excellent source of vitamins A, C, and E
Sodium: 576 mg

Put the onion and peppers into the pan along with the remaining half of the seasoning mixture. Stir and sauté for 2 or 3 minutes more. Add the chicken broth and cook over high heat for 5 to 6 minutes until there is only about ⅓ cup of sauce in the pan. Remove from the heat and stir in the butter.

Evenly distribute the whipped sweet potatoes in the center of each of 4 heated plates. Arrange 2 pieces of pork on each plate and spoon the sauce over it. Serve immediately.

LARRY FORGIONE
....

BRAISED BREAST OF CHICKEN SMOTHERED WITH WHITE BEANS AND GREENS

Serves 4

In this dish, Larry takes advantage of fresh winter greens—some of the only fresh vegetables available during this time of year. He wilts them in a pan with onions and garlic and white beans and serves them with braised chicken breasts. The chef calls for cooked (or canned and drained) white beans. If you cook dried beans for this recipe, figure that ¾ cup of dried beans equals 2 cups cooked.

1 tablespoon extra-virgin olive oil
4 (6-ounce) boneless skinless chicken breasts
Kosher salt (optional)
Few grinds fresh black pepper
1 cup sliced onion
2 teaspoons minced garlic
2 cups cooked or canned and drained white beans, such as cannellini or
   Great Northern
1 tablespoon chopped fresh thyme
4 cups of winter greens, such as mustard, kale, and Savoy cabbage leaves
1 cup homemade chicken broth (page 193) or low-sodium canned broth

In a large nonstick skillet, heat the olive oil. Season the chicken breasts with salt and pepper and sear them over high heat for 1 to 2 minutes on each side. Remove the chicken from the pan.

Put the onions and garlic into the pan and sauté for 1 minute. Add the white beans, thyme, and the greens and return the chicken to the pan. Add the broth and bring to a boil. Lower the heat to a simmer and cook for 10 minutes. Remove the chicken from the pan and set aside to keep warm.

Nutritional Analysis per serving (no salt added)

Calories: 409
Fat: 8.9 g
Saturated fat: 2.0 g
Cholesterol: 108 mg
Sodium: 310 mg
Good source of fiber and vitamins A and C

(continued)

Raise the heat to high and cook the pan ingredients for 2 to 3 minutes, until the liquid is reduced by half.

Place a chicken breast in the center of each of 4 plates or shallow soup bowls. Spoon the white beans, wilted greens, and any liquid over the chicken and serve immediately.

ALICE WATERS

BEAN SOUP WITH WILTED GREENS AND ROSEMARY OIL

Serves 8

As with many soups, it makes sense to make this one in enough quantity to serve eight, despite the fact that other recipes in the book are designed for four. The soup tastes better when made this way and the leftovers are great. Alice infuses olive oil with fresh rosemary to make an aromatic oil that adds incomparable flavor to the soup. We don't deny it also adds calories, so you can avoid this if you are watching your weight. The soup is still good without the extra oil.

2 cups dried white beans, such as cannellini or Great Northern
5 tablespoons extra-virgin olive oil
3 (4- to 5-inch) sprigs fresh rosemary
1 yellow onion, peeled and diced
3 cloves garlic, peeled and sliced thin
2 bay leaves
1 (4-ounce) piece prosciutto bone with rind or 1 (3-inch) piece slab
    bacon (optional)
1 cup chopped seeded, peeled tomatoes
8 cups homemade chicken broth (page 193) or low-sodium canned broth
1 tablespoon kosher salt
About 2 cups greens (a large handful), such as arugula (rocket), chard,
    or young turnip greens, cut into ½-inch strips, if necessary
Few shards fresh Parmesan cheese

Put the beans in a large pot and add enough water to cover by 2 to 3 inches. Refrigerate for 8 hours or overnight. Drain the beans in a colander and discard the soaking water. Rinse well under running water. (Or use the quick-soaking method; see Note below.)

Make the rosemary oil by heating 4 tablespoons of olive oil in a pan until it is warm to the touch. Strip the leaves from 2 sprigs of rosemary and add them to the oil. Set aside in a warm place for 3 to 4 hours. When ready to use, strain the oil and discard the leaves.

To make the soup, heat the remaining tablespoon of olive oil in a nonreactive 4-quart saucepan over medium heat and add the onion and garlic. Cook for about 5 minutes, until the onion is translucent.

Add the remaining sprig of rosemary, the bay leaves, beans, and prosciutto bone, if desired, and cook for 3 to 4 minutes. Add the tomatoes and cook for another minute.

Add the broth and salt and bring to a boil. Lower the heat to a simmer and cook for about 1¼ hours, stirring occasionally. Add the greens and cook for 20 minutes longer.

To serve, pour the soup into a warm tureen and top with the cheese. Drizzle with the rosemary oil and serve.

Note: To prepare the beans by the quick-soaking method, put the beans in a large pot and add enough water to cover by 2 to 3 inches. Bring the beans and water to a boil, reduce the heat, and simmer for 2 minutes. Remove from the heat, cover, and soak for 1 hour. Drain and discard the soaking water. Rinse well. This eliminates the 8 hours of soaking.

Nutritional Analysis per serving (with 1½ teaspoons oil per serving and 2 tablespoons Parmesan cheese and 1 ounce prosciutto)

Calories: 380
Fat: 14.9 g
Saturated fat: 4.2 g
Cholesterol: 13 mg
Very high in fiber
Good source of vitamin A
Sodium: 1,016 mg

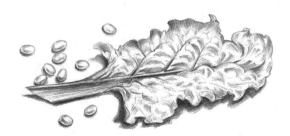

BRAISED DUCK LEGS WITH CELERY ROOT PURÉE
Serves 4

This full-flavored dish is rich, warm, and comforting. The braised duck and creamy purée, topped with a sauce made from the cooking liquid, are perfect on a cold winter's night or for Sunday dinner. Alice prefers Peking duck, also called Chinese duck, for the preparation, but if you cannot buy it, use other duck legs or even chicken legs. When reducing the braising liquid, taste it for saltiness. If too salty, stop the reduction and thicken it with a slurry made by dissolving a teaspoon of potato starch in a small amount of water. Whisk the slurry into the gently boiling liquid until it is incorporated. Also, when making the purée, do not use a food processor or it will turn gluey.

Duck
4 Peking or regular duck legs (drumsticks and thighs)
Kosher salt
Few grinds fresh black pepper
1 tablespoon extra-virgin olive oil
2 tablespoons diced onion
2 tablespoons diced carrot
2 tablespoons diced leek
2 cloves garlic, peeled and sliced thin
Few sprigs fresh thyme
1 bay leaf
½ cup white wine
1½ cups homemade chicken broth (page 193) or low-sodium
    canned broth

Celery Root Purée
3 pounds Yellow Finn potatoes or 2 pounds russet potatoes combined
    with 1 pound red potatoes
1 large celery root (about 8 ounces), cut into 1-inch cubes
¾ cup low-fat milk
3 tablespoons extra-virgin olive oil
½ teaspoon kosher salt
2 grinds fresh black pepper
¼ teaspoon white wine vinegar

To prepare the duck legs, preheat the oven to 375° F.

Season the duck legs lightly with salt and pepper. Heat the olive oil in a skillet over medium-low heat and cook the duck legs for 3 to 4 minutes, turning them several times, until they are golden brown and the fat is rendered. Remove the legs from the pan and set aside.

Scatter the onion, carrot, leek, garlic, thyme, and bay leaf in a small, 3-inch-deep baking dish. Arrange the duck legs, skin side up, on top of the vegetables so that they fit snugly in the dish. Pour in the wine and broth. The liquid should come nearly to the top of the dish. If not, add a little more broth. Cover the dish tightly with foil. Bake for 1 hour.

Meanwhile, make the celery root purée. Peel and quarter the potatoes. Bring 1 gallon of water to a boil and cook the potatoes for about 15 minutes at a medium boil until tender but not crumbly. Drain and lay the potatoes in a shallow dish; let them stand for 15 minutes to dry out.

Bring 2 quarts of water to a boil and cook the celery root for about 20 minutes at a medium boil until tender but not crumbly. Drain in a colander and let the celery root stand for a few minutes to dry out.

Force the potatoes and celery root through a fine mesh food mill or mash them with a potato masher in a large bowl. Add the milk, olive oil, salt, pepper, and vinegar and mix well with a wooden spoon. The purée should be light and fluffy. Keep warm until the duck is done.

Remove the foil from the baking pan. Pour off about half the liquid and reserve it. Most of the skin on the legs should be exposed. Bake uncovered for 30 to 45 minutes, until the skin is nicely browned and the duck meat offers only slight resistance when pierced with a fork or knife. Lift the legs from the liquid and set aside in a warm place, taking care not to tear the skin.

In a saucepan, combine the braising liquid from the baking dish with the reserved liquid. Discard the bay leaf and thyme. Use a ladle to skim any fat from the surface of the liquid. Cook the liquid over medium-high heat for 5 to 6 minutes until reduced by about three quarters. You will have about ¾ cup of sauce.

Reheat the duck legs gently in the sauce. Place them on a platter with the celery root purée. Spoon the sauce around and over the purée and duck legs. Serve immediately.

Nutritional Analysis per serving (duck and sauce only; duck skinned)

Calories: 258
Fat: 16.7 g
Saturated fat: 5.2 g
Cholesterol: 79 mg
Relatively low source of fiber
Good source of vitamin A
Sodium: 310 mg

Nutritional Analysis per serving (celery root puree only)

Calories: 399
Fat: 11.1 g
Saturated fat: 1.8 g
Cholesterol: 1.83 mg
High in fiber and good source of vitamin C
Sodium: 319 mg

ALICE WATERS
....

ROAST LEG OF LAMB WITH EXOTIC SPICES AND YOGURT SAUCE

Serves 4

Alice rubs the lamb with garlic, cumin, fennel seeds, and cayenne and lets it sit for several hours before roasting. The flavors permeate the meat so that after roasting it tastes boldly but not overpoweringly of them. Cool, refreshing yogurt sauce complements the lamb perfectly. You can make the sauce several hours ahead of time.

1 (7-pound) leg of lamb, bone in
1 tablespoon extra-virgin olive oil
2 cloves garlic, peeled and chopped fine
1 scant tablespoon plus ½ teaspoon kosher salt
2½ tablespoons ground cumin
1 tablespoon ground fennel seeds
¼ teaspoon ground red pepper (cayenne)
1 cup plain low-fat yogurt
2 tablespoons finely diced onion
1 teaspoon black pepper
1 teaspoon fresh lemon juice

Rub the lamb with the olive oil and about half the chopped garlic. Combine 1 tablespoon of salt, the cumin, ground fennel seeds, and red pepper. Rub this mixture over the lamb and let the meat stand for 3 to 4 hours at cool room temperature.

Preheat the oven to 375° F.

Put the lamb on a rack set in a shallow roasting pan and roast, uncovered, for about 1 hour and 20 minutes for medium-rare. A meat thermometer inserted near but not touching the bone should read 125 to 130° F.

Nutritional Analysis per serving (without meat drippings)

Calories: 426
Fat: 18 g
Saturated fat: 5.6 g
Cholesterol: 155 mg
Moderate source of fiber
Sodium: 1,464 mg

While the lamb is roasting, mix together the yogurt, onion, black pepper, remaining garlic, the ½ teaspoon of salt, and the lemon juice. Refrigerate until ready to use.

Remove the lamb from the oven and let it rest for 10 minutes before carving into thin slices. Arrange the slices on a warm platter and serve. Pass the yogurt sauce separately.

JIMMY SCHMIDT
....

MAHIMAHI WITH GRAPEFRUIT AND GINGER

Serves 4

Cooking fish in parchment is an excellent way to ensure that it is flavorful and moist without adding fats. Cooking parchment, available in many grocery stores, is as handy to have on hand as waxed paper and aluminum foil. Serving the fish is exceptionally dramatic: Set the puffed-up packet on each plate and invite your guests to open them at the table. The aroma that pours forth as the packets are opened is intoxicating. But warn everyone to beware of the hot steam that accompanies the aroma. You may, if you wish, open the parchment packets in the kitchen and plate the fish there before serving.

For this recipe, Jimmy flavors white, flaky mahimahi, a Pacific Ocean fish, with ginger and grapefruit for a truly tasty Pacific Rim–style dish. If your fish store does not have mahimahi, substitute scrod, pompano, sea bass, halibut, or any other firm, white-fleshed fish.

5 to 6 scallions, trimmed
2 ruby red grapefruit
1 (4-ounce) piece fresh ginger
1 cup sugar
4 (5-ounce) mahimahi fillets
Pinch hot red pepper flakes
4 cups homemade vegetable broth (page 194) or low-sodium broth from
    vegetable bouillon cubes
2 tablespoons Angostura bitters
½ cup nonfat yogurt
¼ cup fresh cilantro leaves

To prepare the mahimahi, halve the scallions, dividing the white and green parts. Slice the green parts into julienne and set aside. Chop the white parts and set aside.

Peel the grapefruit and trim the bitter white pith from the peel. Cut the peel into fine julienne. Separate the fruit into perfect grapefruit segments by using a sharp knife to cut the connecting membrane.

To prepare the ginger, first trim the smaller nubs from the knob and peel the gingerroot. Reserve the nubs and the skin for the sauce. Then, with a very sharp knife, thinly slice the gingerroot with the grain (in the same direction as the fibers). Cut the slices into fine julienne.

Bring 4 cups of water to a boil in a saucepan. Add the sugar and return to a simmer. Add the julienned ginger and cook for about 3 minutes, until tender. Drain in a fine sieve.

Nutritional Analysis per serving

Calories: 308
Fat: 5.3 g
Saturated fat: 1.0 g
Cholesterol: 47 mg
High in vitamins A and C
Moderate amount of fiber
Sodium: 180mg

(continued)

Preheat the oven to 400° F.

Cut 4 pieces of parchment paper into 12 × 16-inch sheets. Fold the sheets in half and cut the open side so that they form half-moons. Open the pieces of parchment and lay them out on the countertop. Place 1 fillet of mahimahi on the lower half of each piece of parchment. Position 2 grapefruit segments over each fillet. Set aside the remaining segments. Scatter the grapefruit rind and the julienne of ginger and scallions on top of the fillets. Sprinkle each with a bit of hot pepper flakes. Fold the top section of parchment over the mahimahi.

Begin to seal the parchment packages at the seam: Fold a ¼ × 1½-inch section of parchment upward and over, and crease to hold. Repeat this folding procedure, and slightly overlap the end of the previous fold to create a tight overlapping seal around the entire open edge of the parchment. Place the parchment pouches on a baking sheet.

Meanwhile, combine the vegetable broth and the reserved chopped scallions in a medium saucepan and bring to a boil over medium-high heat. Cook for about 10 minutes, until the liquid is reduced to 1 cup. Add the ginger peels and trimmings and continue cooking for another 4 minutes or until the liquid is reduced to ½ cup. Remove from the heat and strain through a fine sieve into a small skillet. Discard the solids. Season to taste with the bitters and a pinch of hot pepper flakes, if you desire. Add the remaining grapefruit segments and bring to a simmer. Immediately turn off the heat and gently whisk in the yogurt. Transfer to a sauce bowl and keep warm.

Put the baking sheet holding the parchment pouches in the oven and cook for about 8 minutes, until the parchment is puffed. Serve immediately, one parchment pouch to a plate. Open the pouches at the table. Pass the sauce and cilantro on the side.

JIMMY SCHMIDT

STEAMED MUSSELS WITH SAFFRON AND SPICY COUSCOUS
Serves 4

When you make the couscous, adjust the spices to suit your own tastes. Jimmy infuses the broth with spices before adding couscous to the pot for even distribution of flavors. He prefers New Mexican chili powder, but any high-quality ground chile peppers will work well. Just don't use run-of-the-mill chili seasoning—its flavor is not as good. While the recipe instructs you to mold the couscous in ramekins for a pretty presentation, it is acceptable to scoop it from the pot and mound it in the soup bowls. The couscous is delicious on its own as a side dish, too.

Saffron is a delicate spice that adds a distinctive if subtle flavor to the mussels. It is most easily found in specialty markets, although many supermarkets carry it. A generous pinch will flavor the mussels very nicely. And, finally, for this recipe, you will need about two quarts of mussels (about three pounds).

Couscous
1½ cups homemade vegetable broth (page 194) or low-sodium broth from
    vegetable bouillon cubes
1 teaspoon chili powder or hot Hungarian paprika
1 teaspoon ground cumin
Kosher salt
Few grinds fresh black pepper
2 tablespoons extra-virgin olive oil
1 cup couscous
½ cup minced scallion greens

Steamed Mussels
4 dozen unshucked mussels
2 cups dry white wine, preferably Sauvignon Blanc
1 cup finely diced shallots
4 cloves garlic, peeled and minced
Generous pinch saffron threads
1 teaspoon kosher salt
Freshly ground black pepper

To make the couscous, bring the vegetable broth to a boil in a medium saucepan. Add the chili powder, cumin, a pinch of salt, and the pepper. Cover and take from the heat.

Heat the olive oil in a large skillet over medium-high heat. Add the couscous and stir for 3 to 4 minutes, until hot. Remove the skillet from the heat, add the seasoned broth, and stir.

Let the couscous stand for about 5 minutes to absorb the broth and swell until no liquid remains. Stir in the scallion greens and season to taste with salt and pepper. Keep warm in 250° F oven until serving.

Wash the mussels under cold running water and scrub with a coarse brush to remove any dirt. Do not submerge the mussels in fresh water. Press lightly on any open mussels and discard any that do not close up. Remove the beards by pulling gently with your fingers or a clean needle-nose pliers. Hold the mussels in a colander in the sink covered with a wet paper or kitchen towel.

Combine the white wine with 2 cups of water, the shallots, garlic, saffron, salt, and a generous amount of black pepper in a large nonreactive pot with a tight-fitting lid. Place a steamer basket in the pot. Add the mussels and cover the pot. Bring to a boil over medium-high heat and cook for about 5 minutes, until the mussels open. Remove from the heat. Discard any mussels that have not opened.

To serve, pack the couscous into four 1-cup ramekins or soufflé dishes and invert each one in the center of a shallow soup bowl. Gently lift the ramekin to leave a molded cylinder of couscous. Arrange the opened mussels around each portion of couscous. Ladle the broth from the pot over the mussels, avoiding any grit at the bottom of the pot. Serve immediately.

Nutritional Analysis per serving (with no added salt in the couscous)

Calories: 475
Fat: 11.8 g
Saturated fat: 1.9 g
Cholesterol: 48 mg
High source of fiber and good source of vitamin A
Sodium: 826 mg

Nutritional Analysis per serving (couscous only, no added salt):

Calories: 281
Fat: 7.6 g
Saturated fat: 1.05 g
Cholesterol: 0 mg
High source of fiber
Sodium: 35mg

JIMMY SCHMIDT
....

BRAISED VEAL SHANKS WITH CELERIAC AND MUSTARD

Serves 4

A root vegetable that tastes like celery, celeriac (also called celery root or knob celery) is marketed in the fall and winter months and resembles a round horseradish root. Select a root that is firm and white inside (you may have to rub away dirt to determine the whiteness). Veal shanks are cut from the shins and are best suited to moist, slow braising—just as Jimmy instructs here in this aromatic, full-bodied stew.

1 large celeriac, or celery root
2 tablespoons mustard seeds
2 tablespoons canola oil
4 (12- to 14-ounce) lean veal shanks, trimmed of all fat
12 shallots, peeled
8 cups homemade vegetable broth (page 194) or low-sodium broth from
    vegetable bouillon cubes
Kosher salt (optional)
Few grinds fresh black pepper
3 bay leaves
1 bunch parsley stems
1 tablespoon chopped fresh thyme
¼ cup coarse-grain mustard
¼ cup snipped fresh chives
4 sprigs parsley, for garnish

Trim the celeriac, shape it evenly with a paring knife, and set aside. Spread the mustard seeds in a small skillet and toast over medium-high heat for 6 to 7 minutes, until slightly browned and fragrant. Transfer the seeds to a bowl or plate to cool completely. Set aside.

Preheat the oven to 375° F.

Heat the oil in a large, heavy ovenproof skillet or Dutch oven over medium-high heat. Add the veal shanks and cook for about 3 minutes without turning until seared and browned. Turn the veal shanks on their sides and continue browning. Repeat until all the surfaces have been seared and browned. Remove to a plate and set aside.

> *Nutritional Analysis per serving (without added salt)*
>
> *Calories: 433*
> *Fat: 17.1 g*
> *Saturated fat: 3.1 g*
> *Cholesterol: 146 mg*
> *Moderate amount of fiber*
> *Sodium: 495 mg*
> *High in vitamin A*

To the fat remaining in the skillet, add the peeled whole shallots and cook for about 3 minutes, turning, until lightly browned on all sides. Drain the shallots in a colander to remove any remaining oil.

Return the shanks and shallots to the skillet. Add the vegetable broth and the celeriac and return the skillet to the heat. Season to taste with salt and pepper. Add the bay leaves, parsley stems, and thyme. Bring to a simmer. Cover the skillet by laying aluminum foil, shiny side down, directly on the surface of the broth. Crimp the foil around the skillet to create a good seal. Set the skillet on the lower rack of the oven and bake for about 1 hour and 45 minutes, until the veal is tender. This is determined by inserting a skewer into the meat. When it passes through with no resistance, the veal is done. Remove the skillet from the oven and allow to cool slightly before proceeding.

Remove the celeriac and cut it into large strips. Save about ¼ cup of the irregular trimmings for the sauce. Set aside the sliced celeriac in a small bowl with a little broth to keep it moist.

Remove 2 cups of the liquid from the skillet and strain through a fine sieve into a small saucepan. Bring to a simmer over medium heat and cook for about 5 minutes, until reduced to ½ cup. Remove from the heat and transfer to a blender with the celeriac trimmings. Purée until smooth. Stir in the mustard and chives and season to taste with salt and pepper.

Place 1 veal shank in the center of a shallow soup bowl or serving plate. Arrange the shallots and celeriac strips on top of and around each one. Spoon the mustard sauce over the shanks and vegetables. Sprinkle the toasted mustard seeds over and around the shanks. Garnish each with a sprig of parsley and serve.

JIMMY SCHMIDT

SWORDFISH WITH CORIANDER AND CHIVES
Serves 4

This full-flavored broiled fish is served with a light yogurt-chive sauce. Toasting the coriander seeds releases their intense flavor; the coriander combines with cracked peppercorns to form a crust on the fish.

2 tablespoons coriander seeds
1 tablespoon cracked black peppercorns
4 (5- to 6-ounce) swordfish steaks, trimmed of skin and fat
1 cup dry vermouth
½ cup snipped fresh chives
2 tablespoons low-fat or nonfat plain yogurt
Kosher salt (optional)
4 sprigs parsley, for garnish

Spread the coriander seeds in a small skillet and place over medium-high heat for 3 to 4 minutes until aromatic. Allow to cool. Grind in a spice grinder, small food processor, or coffee grinder until coarse. Alternatively, crush the seeds with a mallet or the back of a sauté pan. Mix the ground coriander seeds with the peppercorns in a small bowl.

(continued)

Preheat the broiler.

Lay the swordfish steaks on a work surface. Divide the coriander and peppercorns evenly among the steaks and gently press onto the top surfaces to adhere. Lay the steaks, spice side up, in an oven-proof skillet. Add the vermouth.

Broil the swordfish for about 6 minutes (depending on thickness) until opaque and beginning to flake. Remove the fish from the skillet and set aside to keep warm.

Set the skillet over high heat, add the chives, and bring to a boil. Immediately remove from the heat. Whisk in the yogurt until the sauce is creamy. Season to taste with salt.

Put the swordfish steaks on a platter or four serving plates and spoon the sauce around them. Garnish with parsley and serve immediately.

Dessert

JIMMY SCHMIDT
....

CRANBERRY AND ORANGE SOUFFLÉ

Serves 6 to 8

Soufflés are light, airy confections that rise to glorious heights, inflated by nothing more complicated than beaten egg whites. Why, then, are so many home cooks wary of them? Fear of falling, no doubt. To avoid this culinary embarrassment, don't be tempted to peer in the oven door while the soufflé is baking. Don't open it even a tiny crack. Busy yourself instead getting the serving plates and garnishes ready. As soon as the soufflé is done, take it from the oven and serve it. Soufflés wait for no one. Jimmy developed this seductively tangy dessert for wintertime parties, taking full advantage of the ripe cranberries and juicy oranges available in the markets. It serves more than four because, quite frankly, it's easier to make a soufflé of this size than a smaller version. That's okay. This dessert is so low in fat and calories that seconds are acceptable.

2 tablespoons unsalted butter, softened
1 cup plus 1 teaspoon granulated sugar
¾ pound fresh cranberries, washed and stemmed
1¼ cups orange juice
2 teaspoons arrowroot or cornstarch
¼ cup orange-flavored liqueur such as Cointreau or Grand Marnier
2 tablespoons grated orange zest
1 tablespoon pure vanilla extract
8 large egg whites
¼ cup coarsely chopped fresh mint plus 6 to 8 mint sprigs
Confectioners' sugar

Nutritional Analysis per serving (no salt added)

Calories: 251
Fat: 7.2 g
Saturated fat: 1.9 g
Cholesterol: 64 mg
Sodium: 161 mg
Relatively low source of fiber

Preheat the oven to 400° F. Butter an 8-cup soufflé dish and sprinkle the sides and bottom with a little sugar.

In a medium saucepan, combine the cranberries, 1 cup of sugar, and 1 cup of the orange juice. Bring to a simmer over medium-high heat and cook for about 15 minutes, until the cranberries are tender and the liquid thickens.

Whisk the arrowroot with the liqueur and the remaining orange juice in a small bowl. Transfer to a blender and add the cranberries, about half at a time. Blend after each addition until smooth. Or purée the mixture in a food processor. Strain through a fine sieve to remove the seeds. Transfer to a large bowl and add the orange zest and vanilla.

Using an electric mixer set at medium-high speed, beat the egg whites to soft peaks. Fold about a quarter of the whites into the cranberry purée, taking care not to overmix. Fold in the rest of the whites about a quarter at a time.

Spoon half the batter into the prepared soufflé dish. Sprinkle the chopped mint over the batter. Spoon the remaining batter into the dish. Smooth the top with a spatula. Set the soufflé on the lower rack of the oven and bake for about 30 minutes, until the soufflé has risen and the top is light brown. Dust the top with confectioners' sugar strained through a fine sieve.

Using 2 spoons, gently cut through the top of the soufflé and move the spoons straight down to the bottom to scoop up part of the interior as well as some crust for each serving. Garnish each serving with a sprig of mint and serve immediately.

Nutritional Analysis per serving (based on 8 servings)

Calories: 210
Fat: 3.1 g
Saturated fat: 1.8 g
Cholesterol: 7.8 mg
Sodium: 57 mg
Relatively low source of fiber

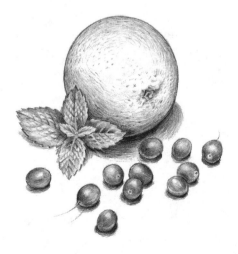

ALICE WATERS
. . . .

PEARS POACHED IN MARSALA

Serves 4

Poached winter pears are a classic dessert. In this recipe, Alice poaches them in sweet Marsala wine with just a hint of orange. Be sure to use nice ripe pears that are not too soft. When figuring how much wine to buy, remember that a liter bottle of Marsala holds just over four cups.

4 cups sweet Marsala wine
½ cup sugar
1 2-inch piece orange zest
4 pears, such as Bosc, Bartlett, or Red Bartlett

Combine the wine, sugar, and orange zest with 3 cups of water in a large saucepan. Bring to a boil, stirring occasionally to dissolve the sugar. Reduce to a low simmer.

Core the pears from the bottom, using an apple corer or sharp knife. Leave the stems intact. Slice the bottom of the pears so that they can sit upright. Using a small sharp knife, peel the pears by stroking down from the top to the bottom in a single motion, if possible. This makes the pears look pretty.

Drop the pears gently into the simmering liquid and raise the heat to medium. Poach for about 25 minutes, turning several times, until they can be pierced easily with a wooden skewer or kitchen knife. Remove the pan from the heat and let the pears cool to room temperature in the liquid.

Lift the pears from the poaching liquid and set aside. Cook the poaching liquid over medium-high heat for about 10 minutes until reduced to 1 cup. It should be a light, sweet syrup that is not too intense. If necessary, cut the sweetness with a little added water.

Arrange the pears on a platter and pour the syrup over them. Serve immediately.

*Nutritional Analysis
per serving*

*Calories: 390
Fat: 0.8 g
Saturated fat: 0.5 g
Cholesterol: 0 mg
Sodium: 11 mg
Good source of fiber*

LARRY FORGIONE
....

BAKED PUMPKIN AND WALNUT PUDDING

Serves 4

As a general rule, the walnuts available by early winter (holiday time) are as fresh as any you can buy all year long. Nuts sold in the spring, summer, and early fall are often left over from the previous year's harvest, but by December the new crop is firmly in place in the market. This dessert comes under the category of sophisticated comfort food.

3 tablespoons unsalted butter, melted, plus 1 teaspoon to coat pan
1 cup plus 1 tablespoon sugar
½ cup chopped walnuts
1 cup unsweetened pumpkin purée
2 large eggs
1⅓ cups all-purpose flour
1 teaspoon baking soda
1 teaspoon baking powder
½ teaspoon ground cinnamon
½ teaspoon grated nutmeg
½ teaspoon salt
1⅓ cups buttermilk
Whipped cream for topping, optional

Preheat the oven to 350° F. Lightly butter a 2-quart square baking dish and sprinkle with a little sugar to coat.

Spread the chopped nuts in a single layer on a baking sheet and toast for 6 to 8 minutes, until fragrant and lightly browned. Transfer to a plate to cool completely.

In a large bowl, combine the pumpkin, 1 cup of sugar, and 2 tablespoons of the melted butter. Add the eggs and beat with an electric mixer set at medium speed for 2 to 3 minutes, until smooth.

Nutritional Analysis per serving (without whipped cream)

Calories: 614
Fat: 21.3 g
Saturated fat: 7.3 g
Cholesterol: 132 mg
Moderate amount of fiber and vitamin A
Sodium: 698 mg

Stir together the flour, baking soda, baking powder, cinnamon, nutmeg, and salt. Add this mixture to the pumpkin batter, alternating with the buttermilk, while mixing at low speed just until combined after each addition. Stir in the toasted walnuts.

Pour the pudding into the baking dish. Place in a shallow roasting pan and pour boiling water into the roasting pan to a depth of about 1 inch. Bake in the center of the oven about 40 minutes, until the pudding is nearly firm in the center when it's gently jiggled. Remove from the oven and sprinkle with the remaining tablespoon of sugar.

Serve immediately with whipped cream, if desired.

BASIC
RECIPES

JIMMY SCHMIDT
....

CHICKEN BROTH

Makes about 10 cups

4 pounds meaty chicken bones, skin removed
2 large onions, diced
2 large carrots, diced
1 large leek, diced
2 bunches fresh parsley stems
2 bay leaves
2 teaspoons black peppercorns
1 sprig fresh thyme

Combine 1 gallon (4 quarts) of water and the chicken bones in a large stock pot. Bring to a simmer over medium heat, skim the surface, and add the remaining ingredients. Return to a gentle simmer, partially cover, and cook for 5 hours, adding more water if necessary to keep the ingredients covered.

Strain through a fine sieve, cool slightly, and refrigerate. Skim off the fatty stock that rises to the surface. The broth will keep in the refrigerator for up to 3 days if well covered. It will keep in the freezer for up to 1 month.

Nutritional Analysis per 1-cup serving:

Calories: Approximately 30
Fat: <1 g
Saturated fat: <1 g
Cholesterol: <5 mg
Sodium: 20 mg
Relatively low source of fiber

JIMMY SCHMIDT

VEGETABLE BROTH
Makes about 6 cups

3 large leeks, washed and diced
3 large onions, diced
1 cup chopped shallots
2 large carrots, diced
3 cups dry white wine
1 bunch parsley stems
2 bay leaves
2 tablespoons black peppercorns

Combine the vegetables with 3 quarts of water and the wine in a large stock pot. Bring to a simmer over medium heat, skim the surface, and add the parsley stems, bay leaves, and peppercorns. Return to a gentle simmer, partially cover, and cook for 4 hours, adding more water if necessary to keep the ingredients covered.

Strain through a fine sieve, cool slightly, and refrigerate until ready to use. The broth will keep in the refrigerator for up to 5 days if well covered. It will keep in the freezer for up to 1 month.

*Nutritional Analysis
per 1-cup serving:*

*Calories: 30
Fat: <1 g
Saturated fat: 0 g
Cholesterol: 0 mg
Sodium: 13 mg
Relatively low source
of fiber*

JIMMY SCHMIDT
....

FISH BROTH

Makes about 8 cups

5 pounds lean fresh salmon or other fish heads and frames
4 cups dry white wine
1 large leek, washed and diced, white and green parts
2 large onions, diced
1 large carrot, diced
1 bunch parsley stems
2 bay leaves
2 tablespoons black peppercorns

Wash the fish heads and frames under running water until the water runs clear. Put the fish heads and frames, 4 quarts of water, and the wine in a large stock pot. Bring to a simmer over medium heat, skim the surface, and add the vegetables, parsley stems, bay leaves, and peppercorns. Return to a gentle simmer, partially cover, and cook for 45 minutes, adding more water if necessary to keep the ingredients covered.

Strain through a fine sieve and refrigerate until ready to use. Skim off fat before using.

Nutritional Analysis per 1-cup serving:

Calories: Approximately 35
Fat: <1 g
Saturated fat: <1 g
Cholesterol: <5 mg
Sodium: 20 mg
Relatively low source of fiber

JIMMY SCHMIDT

GARLIC AND HERB FOCACCIA BUNS
Makes 4 buns

Sourdough Starter
½ teaspoon active dry yeast
½ cup water at 100° F
1 teaspoon cider vinegar
1¼ cups all-purpose flour

Focaccia Dough
½ teaspoon active dry yeast
½ teaspoon sugar
1 tablespoon warm water
1½ teaspoons chopped fresh garlic
1 tablespoon chopped scallions
1½ teaspoons chopped flat-leaf parsley
½ teaspoon salt
1½ teaspoons coarsely ground fresh black pepper
1¼ cups all-purpose flour
1 large egg yolk
¼ cup milk

To make the sourdough starter, combine the yeast, water, and vinegar in a medium bowl. Stir in the flour and cover the bowl with plastic wrap. Set aside for about 1 hour at room temperature until foamy.

To make the bread, combine the yeast, sugar, and water in a large bowl and let sit for about 10 minutes until foamy. Add the sourdough starter and mix well. Add the garlic, scallions, parsley, salt, and pepper.

Nutritional Analysis per bun:

Calories: 310
Fat: 2.4 g
Saturated fat: 0.7 g
Cholesterol: 54 mg
Sodium: 278 mg
Moderate source of fiber

Add the flour and mix until the dough forms a ball. Transfer the dough to a lightly floured work surface and knead for about 8 minutes until smooth and elastic.

Divide the dough into 4 balls of equal size. Shape each into a 6-by-3-inch, slightly flattened oval bun. Transfer all 4 to a parchment-lined baking sheet. Let rise at warm room temperature (about 72° F.) for about 45 minutes until doubled in size.

Preheat the oven to 375° F.

Mix the egg yolk and milk in a small bowl and use to brush the tops of the buns. Leave the buns on the parchment paper and baking sheet and bake on the lower rack of the oven for about 15 to 20 minutes until golden. Lift from the parchment and cool on a wire rack.

A LICE W ATERS
·····················

PESTO

Makes about ¹/₂ cup

1 large clove garlic
Pinch salt
1 cup finely chopped fresh basil
3 tablespoons extra-virgin olive oil
1 heaping tablespoon grated Parmesan cheese (optional)
2 grinds fresh black pepper

Pound the garlic clove and a pinch of salt in a mortar with a pestle until it becomes a smooth paste. Add the basil leaves, a few tablespoons at a time, pounding and working them into a course paste. As the basil mixture becomes thick and dry, add the olive oil, a little at a time. Continue grinding until the mixture becomes a thick, smooth paste and all the olive oil is absorbed. Add the cheese, if desired, and the pepper and mix well with a rubber spatula.

Note: This recipe may be doubled. To make in a food processor, put the garlic and salt in the workbowl fitted with the metal blade and process just until mixed. Add the basil leaves, a few tablespoons at a time, pulsing the processor until the mixture is thick and dry. With the processor running, add the oil in a slow, steady stream until the mixture becomes a thick, smooth paste and all the oil is absorbed. Add the cheese, if desired, and the pepper and mix well with a rubber spatula.

Nutritional Analysis per tablespoon (including Parmesan cheese):

Calories: 54
Fat: 5.6 g
Saturated fat: 1 g
Cholesterol: 1 mg
Sodium: 45 mg
Relatively low source of fiber

Two-Week
Menu Plan

We have assembled two weeks of menus incorporating selected examples of the chefs' recipes into everyday eating patterns. The purpose of these menus is not to dictate specifically what foods you should eat on a day-to-day basis, but instead to give you some idea of how dishes such as those supplied by Alice Waters, Jimmy Schmidt, and Larry Forgione can fit into a daily (or weekly) menu without disrupting a fat-budgeting plan. The amount of calories in most of the daily menus total less than 2,500 with fewer than 60 g of fat. This provides leeway for eating a little more fat one day than the next, for a glass of wine or mixed drink, and for an impulsive ice cream cone, slice of cake, hamburger, or candy bar now and then. We have assumed that most people will not use special recipes from the three chefs for breakfast or lunch during the week and have limited these to weekends. However, any of these can be substituted for a usual breakfast or lunch. One of the chefs' recipes is suggested for each dinner during the two-week plan. Many of the lunch recipes may also be suitable for dinner—these can be substituted.

The following menus were not assembled by the chefs. The meals were put together with the assistance of a nutritionist to reflect what everyday Americans actually eat. Use your common sense to modify these menus to meet your own likes and dislikes. Review the Substitute Recipes lists (*A* and *B*) beginning on page 210. Each recipe in the menu plan is followed by the letter *A* or *B* to indicate which recipe list a substitute can be chosen from. These alternative recipes for the ones in the daily menus are in the same general ballpark as far as calories and fat and can be substituted without much change in the daily totals. Remember that the total calories, fat, and cholesterol contents of the menus in the two-week plan are approximate, since ingredients and choices may vary. However, those listed should give you a good idea of how to budget the food items. Throughout the menus, we suggest drinking coffee, tea, diet beverages, and an occasional alcoholic drink with your meals. For more information on the exact calorie counts of alcoholic and other beverages, turn to Table E at the end of this chapter. In addition, Tables A through D list foods that provide relatively large amounts of antioxidant vitamins and fiber. Keep them in mind when planning your weekly menus.

The following menu plan is designed to maintain weight for a 5-foot 5-inch middle-aged woman weighing 125 pounds or a 6-foot man weighing 175 pounds. It includes an average daily intake of 2,000 to 2,500 calories; 50 to 60 g of total fat (15 to 20 g of saturated fat), and an average of less than 250 mg of cholesterol.

Altering the Two-Week Plan

What about people other than those we used as examples: the 5-foot 5-inch woman and 6-foot man who can eat between 1,900 and 2,300 calories a day and not gain or lose weight? How can you adjust the two-week plan to lose weight or to maintain your current weight if your body is significantly different from our two models?

It is not very difficult. Review Table 1 on page 15, which provides you with the calorie count to maintain your weight, and adjust your calorie intake up or down accordingly. If you are a person who requires fewer than 2,000 calories a day, omit a slice of toast, have a smaller portion, or give up desserts a few times a week. On the other hand, if your calorie requirements are more than 2,500 a day, you can be a little more liberal than outlined in the plan and can add fruits, grains, breads, and low-fat dairy products to your daily menus.

Monday

BREAKFAST

1 (4-ounce) glass of orange or grapefruit juice
1 cup corn flakes, raisin bran, Grape-Nuts, etc
1 banana
Coffee with 1 teaspoon sugar and 1 percent milk, or other hot beverage

CALORIES: 400
FAT: 4 g
SATURATED FAT: 2 g
CHOLESTEROL: 10 mg

LUNCH

Tuna or chicken salad sandwich on hard roll or toast with lettuce and tomato (add a small amount of mayonnaise, if desired)
1 apple
Diet beverage, coffee, or tea

CALORIES: 435
FAT: 12 g
SATURATED FAT: 2 g
CHOLESTEROL: 15 mg

DINNER

Larry Forgione's Braised Breast of Chicken Smothered with White Beans and Greens (recipe on page 175) B
1 dinner roll or rye or wheat bread
1 teaspoon margarine or a little olive oil
1 (5-ounce) glass of white wine
3 graham crackers or gingersnaps
Tea or coffee

CALORIES: 744
FAT: 18 g
SATURATED FAT: 4 g
CHOLESTEROL: 110 mg

COMMENTS: Today was a good day. No reason to cut back or think about fat budgeting tomorrow. You have kept total calories below 2,000, fat calories below 25 percent of the total, saturated fat below 7 percent of the total, and cholesterol well below 250 mg.

DAY'S TOTAL
CALORIES: 1,579
FAT: 34 g (306 fat calories)
SATURATED FAT: 8 g (72 saturated fat calories)
CHOLESTEROL: 135 mg

Tuesday

BREAKFAST

1 (4-ounce) glass of grapefruit or orange juice
1 English muffin or bagel with 1 tablespoon jam or margarine
Coffee with 1 teaspoon sugar and 1 percent milk, or other hot beverage

CALORIES: 250
FAT: 2 g
SATURATED FAT: 1 g
CHOLESTEROL: 1 mg

LUNCH

1 (2-ounce) hot dog (normal-sized) on a bun with mustard, sauerkraut, and relish
½ cup coleslaw
Diet beverage
1 Milky Way bar or other candy bar

CALORIES: 650
FAT: 35 g
SATURATED FAT: 13 g
CHOLESTEROL: 45 mg

DINNER

Jimmy Schmidt's Roasted Beets, Endive, and Frisée Salad (recipe on page 160) A
Jimmy Schmidt's Mahimahi with Grapefruit and Ginger (recipe on page 181) A
Baked potato with 1 teaspoon tub margarine and 2 tablespoons reduced-fat sour cream
1 cup steamed broccoli and cauliflower
1 dinner roll with 1 teaspoon tub margarine
1 cup vanilla ice cream
Coffee or tea

CALORIES: 1,100
FAT: 35 g
SATURATED FAT: 11 g
CHOLESTEROL: 95 mg

COMMENTS: Although you may not have exceeded the total calorie intake, you have eaten too much fat. No guilt feelings necessary! Just watch yourself for the next day or two. (Of course, next time you could substitute sorbet or low-fat yogurt for the ice cream.)

DAY'S TOTAL
CALORIES: 2,000
FAT: 72 g (648 fat calories)
SATURATED FAT: 25 g (225 saturated fat calories)
CHOLESTEROL: 141 mg

Wednesday

BREAKFAST

*4-ounce glass orange or grape-
fruit juice, or orange slices or
½ cantaloupe*
*1 blueberry or bran muffin or
1 bagel with 1 teaspoon tub
margarine*
1 cup 1 percent or skim milk
*Coffee with 1 teaspoon sugar
and 1 percent milk, or other
hot beverage*

CALORIES: 450
FAT: 12 g
SATURATED FAT: 4 g
CHOLESTEROL: 35 mg

LUNCH

*3 ounces turkey on hard roll,
rye bread, or pita bread with
mustard, lettuce, and tomato*
Carrot or celery sticks
1 apple
Diet beverage, coffee, or tea

CALORIES: 360
FAT: 4 g
SATURATED FAT: 1 g
CHOLESTEROL: 35 mg

DINNER

*Alice Waters' Roast Leg of
Lamb with Exotic Spices and
Yogurt Sauce (recipe on page
180) B*
1 cup steamed rice
½ cup peas with pearl onions
*Alice Waters' Pears Poached in
Marsala (recipe on page
188) A*
Coffee, tea, or other beverage

CALORIES: 1,100
FAT: 20 g
SATURATED FAT: 6 g
CHOLESTEROL: 155 mg

COMMENTS: You have made up for some of the excesses of yesterday, but watch yourself tomorrow and Friday, just to make sure.

DAY'S TOTAL
CALORIES: 1,910
FAT: 36 g (324 fat calories)
SATURATED FAT: 11 g (99 satu-
rated fat calories)
CHOLESTEROL: 225 mg

Thursday

BREAKFAST

*1 (4-ounce) glass of orange
juice*
1 bagel
*2 tablespoons reduced-fat
cream cheese or margarine
(You could have your favorite cold cereal instead of a
bagel and cream cheese.)*
*Coffee with 1 teaspoon sugar
and 1 percent milk, or other
hot beverage, or 1 (8-ounce)
glass of 1 percent or skim
milk*

CALORIES: 400
FAT: 7 g
SATURATED FAT: 4 g
CHOLESTEROL: 18 mg

LUNCH

*Mixed salad topped with 3
ounces grilled, skinless teri-
yaki chicken or 3 ounces
chicken salad and 2 tablespoons low-calorie dressing*
Small roll
Fresh fruit
Diet beverage, tea, or coffee

CALORIES: 494
FAT: 10 g
SATURATED FAT: 2 g
CHOLESTEROL: 75 mg

DINNER

*Tossed green salad with 1 table-
spoon low-calorie Italian
dressing or oil and vinegar*
*Larry Forgione's Honey-Glazed
Grouper (recipe on page 173)
A*
2 small boiled red potatoes
*½ cup steamed green and yel-
low squash with 1 teaspoon
tub margarine*
*1 slice rye or wheat bread with
margarine or olive oil*
*3 reduced-fat cookies (or gin-
gersnaps or graham crackers)*
*1 (5-ounce glass) of wine or
diet beverage*

CALORIES: 850
FAT: 28 g
SATURATED FAT: 8 g
CHOLESTEROL: 75 mg

COMMENTS: Not bad. You've eaten well and you are still well
under the budget for fat. If you examine the numbers for the last
three days, you will see that you are right on target, with just
about 25 percent of total calories coming from fat.

DAY'S TOTAL
CALORIES: 1,744
FAT: 45 g (405 fat calories)
SATURATED FAT: 14 g (126 satu-
rated fat calories)
CHOLESTEROL: 168 mg

Friday

BREAKFAST
Orange or grapefruit slices, or 4-ounce orange or grapefruit juice
1 cup bran flakes, shredded wheat, Grape-Nuts, or raisin bran cereal with 1 percent or skim milk
Coffee with 1 teaspoon sugar and 1 percent milk, or other hot beverage, or 1 (8-ounce) glass of skim milk

CALORIES: 300
FAT: 4 g
SATURATED FAT: 2 g
CHOLESTEROL: 10 mg

LUNCH
2 ounces lean roast beef on rye bread with mustard, lettuce, and tomato
1 cup low-fat fruit yogurt
1 orange or apple
Diet beverage, coffee, or tea

CALORIES: 550
FAT: 8 g
SATURATED FAT: 3 g
CHOLESTEROL: 50 mg

DINNER
Alice Waters' Rocket Salad with Baked Ricotta Cheese (recipe on page 98) B
Alice Waters' Summer Minestrone (recipe on page 106) A
Dinner roll with 1 teaspoon tub margarine
1 (5-ounce) glass of wine
Alice Waters' Compote of White Peaches and Nectarines (recipe on page 113) A
Coffee, tea, or diet beverage

CALORIES: 775
FAT: 40 g
SATURATED FAT: 10 g
CHOLESTEROL: 30 mg

COMMENTS: Total calories, cholesterol, and saturated fat are within limits, but the percentage of total fat is a little high.

DAY'S TOTAL
CALORIES: 1,625
FAT: 52 g (468 fat calories)
SATURATED FAT: 15 g (135 saturated fat calories)
CHOLESTEROL: 90 mg

Saturday

BREAKFAST
1 (4-ounce) glass of orange juice
Larry Forgione's Fresh Herb and Spinach Omelet (recipe on page 55) A
2 slices wheat toast with 2 teaspoons tub margarine
1 cup 1 percent milk
Coffee with 1 teaspoon sugar and 1 percent milk, or other hot beverage

CALORIES: 592
FAT: 22 g
SATURATED FAT: 5 g
CHOLESTEROL: 169 mg

LUNCH
Larry Forgione's Roasted Corn and Chanterelle Salad with Autumn Greens (recipe on page 125) A
2 slices French bread with margarine
1/2 cup fruit sorbet
Diet beverage, coffee, or tea

CALORIES: 541
FAT: 21 g
SATURATED FAT: 4 g
CHOLESTEROL: 0 mg

DINNER
1 (5-ounce) mixed drink cocktail
Alice Waters' Endive, Apple, and Walnut Salad (recipe on page 129) A
Larry Forgione's Roast Chicken with Apple-Sage Dressing (recipe on page 145) B
Baked potato with 1 teaspoon tub margarine
1/2 cup steamed green beans
1 cup fresh fruit salad or apple
Diet beverage

CALORIES: 1,456
FAT: 56 g
SATURATED FAT: 21 g
CHOLESTEROL: 171 mg

COMMENTS: Today, your calorie, fat, saturated fat, and cholesterol intakes were all too high—you made up for some of the low-calorie days. But before we panic, let's see how the total week's intake looks after tomorrow.

DAY'S TOTAL
CALORIES: 2,589
FAT: 99 g (891 fat calories)
SATURATED FAT: 30 g (270 saturated fat calories)
CHOLESTEROL: 340 mg

Sunday

BREAKFAST

Jimmy Schmidt's Pear, Parsnip, and Potato Pancakes (recipe on page 158) B
1 cup 1 percent or skim milk
Coffee with 1 teaspoon sugar and 1 percent milk, or other hot beverage

CALORIES: 638
FAT: 11 g
SATURATED FAT: 6 g
CHOLESTEROL: 74 mg

LUNCH

Alice Waters' Pasta with Mushrooms, Fennel, and Thyme (recipe on page 166) B
1 slice Italian bread
1 teaspoon tub margarine
Tossed green salad with 1 to 2 tablespoons reduced-fat blue cheese dressing or oil and vinegar
½ cup fruit salad or apple or pear
Diet beverage

CALORIES: 650
FAT: 9 g
SATURATED FAT: 2 g
CHOLESTEROL: 74 mg

DINNER

Jimmy Schmidt's Vegetable Black Bean Chili (recipe on page 162) A
4 ounces broiled swordfish
½ cup cooked carrots
1 (5-ounce) glass white wine
Jimmy Schmidt's Cranberry and Orange Soufflé (recipe on page 186) A
Coffee with 1 teaspoon sugar and 1 percent milk, or other hot beverage

CALORIES: 760
FAT: 17 g
SATURATED FAT: 5 g
CHOLESTEROL: 160 mg

COMMENTS: Cholesterol intake is high. But you've had a lovely Sunday. Now let's see what the first week's average daily intakes of calories, fat, and cholesterol were.

DAY'S TOTAL
CALORIES: 2,048
FAT: 37 g (333 fat calories)
SATURATED FAT: 13 g (117 saturated fat calories)
CHOLESTEROL: 308 mg

Average Intake per Day for Week 1

COMMENTS: The weekly average is not bad at all (despite the weekend). Total calories average below 2,000 a day. Fat calorie intake is just about 25 percent of total calories, and saturated fat intake is about 8 percent. Daily cholesterol intake is below 250 mg a day. The fat budgeting system is working!

CALORIES: 1,928
FAT: 54 g (486 fat calories)
SATURATED FAT: 17 g (153 saturated fat calories)
CHOLESTEROL: 201 mg

Monday

BREAKFAST
*4-ounce glass orange juice or
1 slice honeydew melon or ½
cantaloupe
3 (4-inch) pancakes (prepared
from a mix)
2 tablespoons maple syrup
1 cup 1 percent or skim milk
Coffee with 1 teaspoon sugar
and 1 percent milk, or other
hot beverage*

CALORIES: 508
FAT: 9 g
SATURATED FAT: 3 g
CHOLESTEROL: 63 mg

LUNCH
*2 ounces turkey breast on rye
bread with mustard, lettuce,
and tomato
1 cup low-fat fruit yogurt or
1 apple or pear
Diet beverage, coffee, or tea*

CALORIES: 541
FAT: 6 g
SATURATED FAT: 2 g
CHOLESTEROL: 33 mg

DINNER
*Tossed green salad with 1 table-
spoon oil and vinegar
Jimmy Schmidt's Pork Chops
with Mustard and Rosemary
(recipe on page 131) B
1 medium baked potato
½ cup cooked beets
1 roll
2 teaspoons tub margarine (divided between potato and
roll)
Diet beverage
Alice Waters' Baked Figs in
Red Wine (recipe on page
153) A
Coffee or tea*

CALORIES: 1,025
FAT: 41 g
SATURATED FAT: 11 g
CHOLESTEROL: 135 mg

COMMENTS: You're off to a reasonably
good start this week. There is some
room to have an apple, pear, or orange
for a snack or a glass of wine instead
of a diet beverage for dinner, without
exceeding the budget by very much.

DAY'S TOTAL
CALORIES: 2,074
FAT: 56 g (504 fat calories)
SATURATED FAT: 16 g (144 satu-
rated fat calories)
CHOLESTEROL: 231 mg

Tuesday

BREAKFAST
*½ grapefruit
2 (4-inch) whole-grain waffles
or whole-grain cereal with
skim or 1 percent milk
2 tablespoons maple syrup
1 teaspoon tub margarine
1 cup 1 percent milk
Coffee with 1 teaspoon sugar
and 1 percent milk, or other
hot beverage*

CALORIES: 523
FAT: 16 g
SATURATED FAT: 6 g
CHOLESTEROL: 90 mg

LUNCH
*Chef's salad with about 1
ounce turkey and 1 ounce
ham
2 tablespoons reduced-calorie
Italian dressing or oil and
vinegar
1 small roll with 1 teaspoon
tub margarine
3 to 4 gingersnaps or graham
crackers
Diet beverage, coffee, or tea*

CALORIES: 417
FAT: 15 g
SATURATED FAT: 3 g
CHOLESTEROL: 25 mg

DINNER
*1 (5-ounce) glass white wine
Alice Waters' Baked Salmon
with Watercress Sauce (recipe
on page 71) A
1 cup steamed rice
½ cup steamed carrots
Jimmy Schmidts' Low-Fat
Chocolate Brownie (recipe on
page 78) with ½ cup low-fat
frozen yogurt A
Coffee or tea*

CALORIES: 969
FAT: 25 g
SATURATED FAT: 6 g
CHOLESTEROL: 135 mg

COMMENTS: No reason to be concerned about today's intake except for the total intake of cholesterol; fat and saturated fat are
okay. (Shrimp contains a lot of cholesterol but is low in fat.)

DAY'S TOTAL
CALORIES: 1,909
FAT: 56 g (504 calories)
SATURATED FAT: 15 g (135
calories)
CHOLESTEROL: 250 mg

Wednesday

BREAKFAST
1 (4-ounce) glass of orange or grapefruit juice
1 scrambled egg
2 slices white or whole wheat toast with margarine
1 tablespoon jelly
Coffee with 1 teaspoon sugar and 1 percent milk

CALORIES: 486
FAT: 17 g
SATURATED FAT: 4 g
CHOLESTEROL: 260 mg

LUNCH
Alice Waters' Provençal Chicken Salad (recipe on page 130) A
2 small graham crackers or gingersnaps
1 cup 1 percent milk, coffee, or tea
Diet beverage

CALORIES: 575
FAT: 17 g
SATURATED FAT: 4g
CHOLESTEROL: 28 mg

DINNER
1 (5-ounce) glass of red wine
Alice Waters' Baked Chanterelles with Garlic Toasts (recipe on page 128) A
Alice Waters' Grilled Steak with Gremolata (recipe on page 138) A
3 boiled new potatoes with 1 teaspoon tub margarine
Sliced tomatoes with 1 tablespoon oil and vinegar
3 reduced-fat cookies or gingersnaps
Coffee, tea, or other beverage

CALORIES: 948
FAT: 27 g
SATURATED FAT: 7.2 g
CHOLESTEROL: 107 mg

COMMENTS: You are above the limit on total fat intake today and way over the limit on cholesterol. Make Thursday a day to cut back.

DAY'S TOTAL
CALORIES: 2,009
FAT: 61 g (549 fat calories)
SATURATED FAT: 15 g (135 saturated fat calories)
CHOLESTEROL: 395 mg

Thursday

BREAKFAST
4-ounce glass orange juice
1 cup Product 19, Special K, or other cold cereal with skim or 1 percent milk
1 banana
1 slice raisin toast with margarine or jam
Coffee with 1 teaspoon sugar and 1 percent milk, or other hot beverage

CALORIES: 503
FAT: 8 g
SATURATED FAT: 3 g
CHOLESTEROL: 10 mg

LUNCH
Small bowl of minestrone soup (low-sodium soup if on a low-salt diet)
6 low-fat crackers
1 apple
Diet beverage, coffee, or tea

CALORIES: 351
FAT: 7 g
SATURATED FAT: 3 g
CHOLESTEROL: 7 mg

DINNER
Mixed greens with 1 tablespoon oil and vinegar
Jimmy Schmidt's Grilled Breast of Chicken with Sweet Corn and Wild Mushroom Salsa (recipe on page 110) B
1 cup cooked barley
Fresh fruit
Diet beverage, coffee, or tea

CALORIES: 760
FAT: 27 g
SATURATED FAT: 5 g
CHOLESTEROL: 96 mg

COMMENTS: Today you are well under your budget—which makes up for yesterday.

DAY'S TOTAL
CALORIES: 1,614
FAT: 42 g (378 fat calories)
SATURATED FAT: 11 g (99 saturated fat calories)
CHOLESTEROL: 113 mg

Friday

BREAKFAST
1 (4-ounce) glass of grapefruit juice
1 cup oatmeal, other hot cereal, or cold cereal with 1 percent or skim milk
1 cup sliced bananas, strawberries, blueberries, or peaches
Coffee with 1 teaspoon sugar and 1 percent milk, or other hot beverage

CALORIES: 422
FAT: 6 g
SATURATED FAT: 2 g
CHOLESTEROL: 11 mg

LUNCH
Tossed salad with 1 tablespoon vinaigrette
2 slices cheese pizza from large pie (plain or with mushrooms—but not pepperoni)
Diet beverage

CALORIES: 645
FAT: 20 g
SATURATED FAT: 7 g
CHOLESTEROL: 35 mg

DINNER
1 (5-ounce) glass of white wine or a cocktail
Larry Forgione's Grilled Veal Chops with Summer Garden Salad (recipe on page 103) A
1 cup prepared wild rice mix (using margarine)
2 to 3 steamed broccoli spears
Diet beverage
Jimmy Schmidt's Nectarine and Blackberry Crisp (recipe on page 117) B
Coffee with 1 teaspoon sugar and 1 percent milk

CALORIES: 1,120
FAT: 31 g
SATURATED FAT: 9 g
CHOLESTEROL: 146 mg

COMMENTS: Your total and saturated fat intakes are at the upper limits of where you want to be. You are still on track. Check out the week's totals after Sunday to see if you may have to be more careful.

DAY'S TOTAL
CALORIES: 2,187
FAT: 57 g (513 fat calories)
SATURATED FAT: 18 g (162 saturated fat calories)
CHOLESTEROL: 192 mg

Saturday

BREAKFAST
1 (4-ounce) glass of orange or grapefruit juice
Jimmy Schmidt's Summer Berry and Maple Pancakes (recipe on page 82) B
1 cup 1 percent milk
Coffee with 1 teaspoon sugar and 1 percent milk, or other hot beverage

CALORIES: 705
FAT: 12 g
SATURATED FAT: 4 g
CHOLESTEROL: 65 mg

LUNCH
3 ounces extra-lean hamburger on bun
Catsup or mustard
1 bunch grapes (about 20), apple, or pear
Diet beverage

CALORIES: 444
FAT: 16 g
SATURATED FAT: 6 g
CHOLESTEROL: 84 mg

DINNER
1 (5-ounce) glass of white wine
Larry Forgione's Swordfish with Charred Tomato Vinaigrette (recipe on page 101) B
1 boiled or baked potato
1 cup steamed carrots, green beans, sugar peas, or broccoli
Larry Forgione's Lemon Angel Food Chiffon (recipe on page 115) B
Coffee with 1 teaspoon sugar and 1 percent milk, or other hot beverage

CALORIES: 1,274
FAT: 42 g
SATURATED FAT: 13 g
CHOLESTEROL: 212 mg

COMMENTS: It's Saturday and you are over budget for cholesterol and fat.

DAY'S TOTAL
CALORIES: 2,423
FAT: 70 g (630 fat calories)
SATURATED FAT: 23 g (207 saturated fat calories)
CHOLESTEROL: 361 mg

Sunday

BREAKFAST

*1 (4-ounce) glass of tomato, or-
ange, or grapefruit juice*
*Larry Forgione's Summer Vege-
table Frittata (recipe on page
84) B*
*1 slice wheat toast with tub
margarine*
*Coffee with 1 teaspoon sugar
and 1 percent milk, or other
hot beverage*

CALORIES: 517
FAT: 18 g
SATURATED FAT: 6 g
CHOLESTEROL: 176 mg

LUNCH

*Jimmy Schmidt's Sweet Pepper,
Eggplant, Tomato, and Arugula Sandwich (recipe on
page 88) B*
½ cup orange sherbet
Diet beverage

CALORIES: 610
FAT: 12 g
SATURATED FAT: 3 g
CHOLESTEROL: 32 mg

DINNER

*Jimmy Schmidt's Spicy Shrimp
with Bitter Greens Salad (recipe on page 99) A*
3 ounces filet mignon
*1 large baked potato with 1
teaspoon tub margarine and
2 tablespoons reduced-fat sour
cream*
*1 cup steamed zucchini and
summer squash*
1 small slice fat-free cake
Diet beverage, coffee, or tea

CALORIES: 812
FAT: 32 g
SATURATED FAT: 8 g
CHOLESTEROL: 118 mg

COMMENTS: Today is also over budget, especially for cholesterol.
You didn't do too well this weekend, but you certainly ate well.
Exercise prudence early next week. Before you get discouraged,
let's see how the daily average works out.

DAY'S TOTAL
CALORIES: 1,939
FAT: 62 g (558 fat calories)
SATURATED FAT: 17 g (153 satu-
rated fat calories)
CHOLESTEROL: 326 mg

Average Intake per Day for Week 2

COMMENTS: Compare this to last week—the numbers are very
close. You are a little high on cholesterol, but total fat and saturated fat are pretty close to target. Once again, clearly, fat budgeting works.

CALORIES: 2,022
FAT: 58 g (519 fat calories)
SATURATED FAT: 16 g (144 satu-
rated fat calories)
CHOLESTEROL: 267 mg

Average Intake per Day for Both Weeks

COMMENTS: You could not possibly say that you have deprived
yourself with this kind of eating. Note that you had some meat
(for lunch or dinner, on three or four days of each week) without
exceeding the desired total fat or cholesterol intake. You have
eaten less red meat than poultry and fish, which is how it should
be.

These menus certainly can be altered. Many people might prefer pasta two or more evenings a week, or might want chicken or
fish more frequently. And that's fine. We simply want to illustrate
that you can eat well and still stay on a low-fat, low-cholesterol
diet. Adjustments can easily be made if you have been advised to
reduce daily cholesterol intake to below 200 mg or saturated fat
to below 7 to 8 percent.

CALORIES: 1,975
FAT: 56 g (504 fat calories—or 26
percent of total)
SATURATED FAT: 17 g (153 saturated fat calories—or 8 percent
of total)
CHOLESTEROL: 234 mg

Substitute Recipes

The following are suggestions for recipe substitutions for the chefs' recipes named throughout the two-week plan. If a recipe is labeled *A*, substitute another recipe from the *A* list. These recipes have approximately the same calorie and fat content (although their sodium and cholesterol may not match), and can be eaten in place of the suggested recipe.

There are numerous other recipes in the book that can be used in place of the suggested recipe or those on the following lists. Simply compare the nutritional values at the end of each recipe and make an appropriate substitution.

A List (These recipes generally have fewer than 350 calories and 15 g of fat)

Breakfast
Alice Waters' Compote of Tangerines and Blood Oranges (recipe on page 53)
Larry Forgione's Warm Apple and Blueberry Compote with Granola and Yogurt (recipe on page 121)

Lunch and Salads
Jimmy Schmidt's Calamari, White Bean, and Red Lentil Ragout (recipe on page 161)
Jimmy Schmidt's Spinach, Roasted Pepper, Onion, and Mâche Salad (recipe on page 132)
Larry Forgione's Chilled Oysters with a Cucumber-Mint Sauce (recipe on page 64)
Larry Forgione's Prosciutto with a Roasted Beet and Fig Salad and a Citrus Dressing
    (recipe on page 127)

Dinner
Alice Waters' Spring Turnip Soup (recipe on page 72)
Alice Waters' Onion and Roasted Pepper Panade (recipe on page 140)
Jimmy Schmidt's Braised Veal Shanks with Celeriac and Mustard (recipe on page 184)
Larry Forgione's Herb-Seared Snapper Fillet with Marinated Cucumber and Tomatoes
    (recipe on page 104)

Dessert
Alice Waters' Strawberry Granita (recipe on page 77)
Larry Forgione's Angel Food Cake (recipe on page 114)

B List (These recipes generally have more than 350 calories and 15 g of fat.)

Lunch and Salads
Alice Waters' Tomato Confit on Toasted Bread with Pesto (recipe on page 89)
Alice Waters' Pasta with Bitter Spring Greens (recipe on page 60)
Jimmy Schmidt's Sea Scallops, Red Peppers, and Marjoram Angel Hair Pasta (recipe on page 87)
Jimmy Schmidt's Shrimp and Sorrel Risotto (recipe on page 62)
Larry Forgione's Warm Chicken Salad with Walnut Sherry Vinaigrette (recipe on page 168)
Larry Forgione's Native Bean Soup (recipe on page 124)

Dinner
Jimmy Schmidt's Chicken Grilled with Citrus, Roasted Garlic, and Artichokes (recipe on page 68)
Jimmy Schmidt's Chile-Rubbed Tuna with Tomatillo Chutney (recipe on page 112)
Jimmy Schmidt's Steamed Mussels with Saffron and Spicy Couscous (recipe on page 182)

Larry Forgione's Grilled Chicken, Forest Mushrooms, and Red Onion Pasta (recipe on page 73)
Larry Forgione's Braised Mahimahi with Fresh Succotash (recipe on page 105)
Larry Forgione's Seared Fillets of Pork with Chili Spices (recipe on page 174)
Alice Waters' Bean Soup with Wilted Greens and Rosemary Oil (recipe on page 176)
Alice Waters' Pasta with Clams, Thyme, and Garlic (recipe on page 139)

Dessert
Larry Forgione's Chocolate Cherry Fudge Cake (recipe on page 76)
Jimmy Schmidt's Baked Pear with Wildflower Honey, Wine, and Vanilla (recipe on page 151)

TABLE 10

CALORIES AND TOTAL FAT CALORIES TO MAINTAIN WEIGHT FOR PEOPLE AT IDEAL (OR ALMOST IDEAL) WEIGHT[1]

	HEIGHT/WEIGHT	TOTAL CALORIES TO MAINTAIN WEIGHT	TOTAL AS FAT CALORIES (APPROXIMATE)[2]
MODERATELY ACTIVE WOMEN	5'1"/105–110 LB	1,575–1,650	400
	5'3"/115–120	1,725–1,800	450
	5'5"/125–130	1,875–1,950	480
	5'7"/135–140	2,025–2,100	520
MODERATELY ACTIVE MEN	5'9"/160–165	2,400–2,475	610
	5'11"/170–175	2,550–2,625	650
	6'1"/180–185	2,700–2,775	690
	6'3"/195–200	2,925–3,000	730

[1] *Remember: To lose weight, reduce calorie content as follows: by 500 calories per day if your target is to lose 1 pound per week; by 1,000 calories per day if your target is to lose 2 pounds per week, or reduce calories by less than that and use up the difference in calories by exercising.*
[2] *To determine the number of grams of fat, divide by 9.*

If You Want to Lose Weight
In the box Sample Calorie Targets for Losing Weight (page 16), we reviewed calorie targets for losing weight and presented two examples. To repeat, let's assume that you were overweight and reduced your total weekly calorie intake by 3,500 calories. You would lose 1 pound. You would also lose 1 pound if you reduced your total weekly calorie intake by 3,000 and burned up an extra 500 calories with exercise. The box Examples of How to Plan a Weight Loss Program gives some specific examples. How does this fit into the Two-Week Menu Plan?

Let's look at Saturday of Week 2. Instead of Larry Forgione's Lemon Angel Food Chiffon without sauce (474 calories), have an apple (70 calories). Omit the hamburger (448 calories) and instead have a tuna salad sandwich (278 calories). As another example, on Friday of Week 1, omit the canned fruit in light syrup (125 calories) and have orange juice (50 calories) instead. Cut back the spaghetti to one cup (180 calories) and forgo Larry Forgione's dessert. Substitute fruit sherbet (135 calories per half cup). Another good way to cut calories is to omit bread whenever possible. Find some of the chef's recipes that have fewer calories than others and substitute as you feel necessary to reduce the calorie totals by the required amount. (And remember, you can lose half a pound one week and one and a half pounds the following week simply by rearranging the menus.)

Examples of How to Plan a Weight Loss Program*

To lose 1 pound a week: Reduce daily calorie intake by about 500 calories/day, or a total of 3,500 calories/week

or

reduce calories by only 300/day and burn up an extra 200 calories/day with exercise. This can be done by: 1) walking at a moderate pace (2 mph) for 1 hour/day; or 2) playing golf (about 200 to 250 calories per hour, for a total of 600 to 800 calories per 18 holes) several times a week. Moderate bicycling, tennis, climbing stairs, dancing, housecleaning, or gardening will also help.

To lose 2 pounds/week: Reduce daily calorie intake by 1,000 calories/day or combine a reduction in calories of 600 to 700 calories/day with an increase in exercise calories of 300 to 400/day. This is not too difficult to accomplish.

An extra 2,000 calories/week can be expended without strenuous workouts. Example:

PLACE	ACTIVITY	APPROXIMATE EXTRA CALORIES USED UP/WK
At home or at work	Climb 2 flights of stairs/day	300
	Walk 1–1½ miles/day (at work, to the train or bus, etc.)	700
At leisure	Walk 4–5 miles/week	300
	Participate in some sport (such as tennis, swimming, biking, or golf) for 1–2 hours/week	700
	Total:	2,000

* *Also see the box Sample Calorie Targets for Losing Weight (page 16).*

What About Eating in Restaurants?

In the world in which we live, more and more people are eating out than ever before. If you have read *Heart-Healthy Cooking for All Seasons,* you have a general idea of the calorie and fat contents of various foods. Use your judgment when eating out.

For dinner: Don't go the whole way. A main course and a salad are often enough, and it's a good idea to ask for the salad dressing "on the side." Limit the number of rolls and pieces of bread you eat. Finish the meal with fruit and coffee. Have dessert only on rare occasions.

Lunch and Fast Foods: Most restaurants have turkey (not turkey roll, if possible), tuna and chicken salad, grilled chicken, and ham that can be eaten in sandwiches. They also often have pasta salads, which are another good choice. Avoid fried foods (including french fries, except on rare occasions) and pies and cakes (again, except on rare occasions). Treat yourself to a hot dog or a burger once in a while, but remember to count it when you figure your daily and weekly totals.

The Morning Coffee Cart: It's tempting, but don't succumb to those doughnuts and Danish every morning. Each one has at least 150 calories and is loaded with fat. If you do indulge now and then, remember to watch yourself for the rest of the day.

TABLE 11
GOOD SOURCES OF VITAMIN A
(in international units)

Sweet potato	1 medium	12,430
Carrot, raw	1 large	10,120
Butternut squash, cooked	½ cup	4,290
Spinach, steamed	3 ounces	2,715
Cantaloupe	¼ melon	2,150
Red pepper, raw	1 medium	2,110
Mango	½ cup	1,605
Vegetarian vegetable soup	1 cup	1,505
Apricot nectar	6 ounces	1,245
V-8 juice	6 ounces	1,060
Collard greens, boiled	½ cup	875
Romaine lettuce	1 cup	730
Pumpkin, fresh, boiled	½ cup	665
Broccoli spears, steamed	2 spears	515
Apricot, fresh	1 medium	460
Tomato, fresh	1 medium	380
Peach, fresh	1 medium	235

Note: The U.S. Recommended Daily Allowance (USRDA) for men = 5,000 IU; for women = 4,000 IU. A balanced diet provides plenty of vitamin A. Vitamin A supplements that supply more than 10,000 IU/day may be dangerous during pregnancy—check with your doctor.

TABLE 12
GOOD SOURCES OF VITAMIN C
(in milligrams)

Grapefruit juice	6 ounces	246
Red pepper, raw	1 medium	141
Orange juice	6 ounces	129
Total cereal	1 cup	70
Green pepper, raw	1 medium	66
Broccoli, steamed	½ cup	62
Cantaloupe	¼ melon	56
Strawberries	½ cup	47
Grapefruit	½ fruit	47
Potato, baked	1 medium	26
Cauliflower	½ cup	25
Tomato, fresh	1 medium	24

Note: The Recommended Daily Allowance (USRDA) for men and women is 60 mg. As you can see, you can get plenty of vitamin C in your daily food.

TABLE 13
GOOD SOURCES OF VITAMIN E
(in milligrams)

Total cereal	1 cup	34.9
Product 19 cereal	1 cup	34.9
Nutri-Grain Wheat cereal	1 cup	11.6
Sunflower seeds, dried	2 tablespoons	9.1
Hazelnuts	1 ounce	7.1
Sunflower oil	1 tablespoon	6.9
Sweet potato	1 medium	5.2
Wheat germ, toasted	2 tablespoons	3.6
Salmon, broiled	4 ounces	2.8
Canola oil	1 tablespoon	2.2
Margarine, tub	1 tablespoon	2.1

Note: 1 mg is equal to approximately 1.51 IU—(Most supplements of Vitamin E are sold in international units.)

The U.S. Recommended Daily Allowance (USRDA) for men = 10 mg (or 15 IU); for women = 8 mg (or 12 IU). You may not be able to get enough Vitamin E in food to be effective as an antioxidant. All of the information on this was obtained with 100 to 400 units a day. Check with your doctor about the possible use of supplements.

TABLE 14
GOOD SOURCES OF FIBER
(in grams)

Wheat bran	2 ounces	23.8
Oat bran	2 ounces	15.7
Rolled oats	1 bowl (6 ounces)	23.6
Corn flakes	1 bowl (6 ounces)	20.7
Grape-Nuts	1 bowl (6 ounces)	22.1
Pinto beans	8 ounces	23.7
White beans	8 ounces	19.6
Kidney beans	8 ounces	23
Lima beans	8 ounces	21.9
Corn	1 ear (4 ounces)	3.7
Sweet potato	1 medium (6 ounces)	4.3
Kale	4 ounces	2.9
Asparagus	about 6 stalks (6 ounces)	2.7
Cucumber	1 medium (4 ounces)	1
Apple	1 medium (4 ounces)	2.3
Orange	1 medium (4 ounces)	2.3
Banana	1 large (4 ounces)	2
Peach	1 medium (4 ounces)	1.6

Note: The recommended intake of fiber for men and women is between 20 and 35 g a day. The foods on this chart are not only good sources of needed fiber; they are also low in fat and none contain cholesterol.

TABLE 15

APPROXIMATE CALORIC CONTENT OF ALCOHOLIC
AND CARBONATED BEVERAGES

Beer 12 ounces	145
Gin, rum, vodka, whiskey, bourbon, rye, scotch, 86 proof 1½ ounces	110
Manhattan 3½ ounces	160
Martini 3½ ounces	180
Champagne 4 ounces	80
Sherry 2 ounces	85
Wines 3½ ounces	130
Carbonated, nonalcoholic (quinine sodas)	90
Ginger ale 8 ounces	70
Root beer 10 ounces	120
Cola 10 ounces	115
Fruit-flavored sodas 10 ounces	130

APPENDIX

YOUR PERSONAL RISK FOR HEART DISEASE
BASED ON CHOLESTEROL LEVELS

Tables 16 and 17 will help to give you an idea of what your real individual or absolute risk of developing heart disease is with increasing levels of cholesterol in your blood. This should help to clarify the debate about what doubling or tripling of the risk for a disease is all about. For example, to be told that with a cholesterol level of 290 your risk of developing a heart attack is double that of someone whose cholesterol level is 200 sounds like a catastrophe. For a forty-year-old woman with a blood cholesterol level of 290 compared to one of 200, the risk is indeed *doubled* to 2 compared to 1—for every *100* persons over a *ten-year* period of time (two cardiac events per 1,000 people compared to one per 1,000 per year; see Table 16). The percentage given (double, or 200 percent) represents the risk based on large population studies. It is called a "relative risk" estimation. A woman with this level of cholesterol may wish to do something about her added risk but should recognize that the absolute individual or personal risk based upon specific numbers— 2 versus 1—while increased, is not that great. In a young woman of about forty, the absolute or individual risk doesn't get too high even with a cholesterol of 290 unless she has two to three other risk factors or actual heart disease—and, of course, if her HDL level is high, the risk of elevated cholesterol is decreased.

Even for a man of forty (Table 17) with no risk factors other than an elevated blood cholesterol of 290, the increased number of potential heart complications is only 3 per 100 people over ten years (6 compared to 3). But let's look at a male with a high blood cholesterol plus high blood pressure and diabetes (risk factors that often go together, along with obesity and a sedentary existence). Here the absolute individual risk is considerably higher, especially when we look at people aged fifty, sixty or older. In older women, the risk is considerably greater than in younger women.

Another point: A man of fifty with a high blood cholesterol level (about 290) who is a smoker and has high blood pressure (two other risk factors) has a relatively high heart attack risk of about 24 for every 100 persons over ten years. Even if he reduces his cholesterol to 200 (a difficult task without medication), the risk will be reduced only to 17/100/ ten years. He must change his other risk factors to have a major impact on his life span.

Tables 18 and 19 will actually help you determine whether you are in a low-, mild- to moderate-, or high-risk category. These are defined as 1) less than a 5 percent chance of having a heart attack in the next 10 years; 2) a 5 to 20 percent chance; or 3) more than a 20 percent chance. These estimates are based on age, gender, and the presence or absence of risk factors in addition to cholesterol levels.

The boxes on the next pages will give you some idea of where you stand and what your absolute heart attack risks are if your blood cholesterol levels are normal, borderline, or high, and if you have other risk factors.

TABLE 16

APPROXIMATE RISK OF SUFFERING HEART DISEASE FOR 100 WOMEN OVER A 10-YEAR PERIOD ACCORDING TO RISK FACTORS*

	AGE 40 SERUM CHOLESTEROL LEVEL (MG/DL)			AGE 50 SERUM CHOLESTEROL LEVEL (MG/DL)			AGE 60 SERUM CHOLESTEROL LEVEL (MG/DL)		
	200	250	290	200	250	290	200	250	290
With no other risk factors	1	1	2	3	5	6	5	6	8
Also is a smoker (S)	2	3	4	6	8	10	8	11	13
Also has high blood pressure	2	3	4	6	8	10	8	11	13
Also has diabetes	3	4	6	8	10	12	10	13	15
With a low HDL (below 35)	3	4	6	9	11	14	11	14	17
With two other risk factors (S and BP↑)	4	6	7	10	13	15	13	17	20
With three other risk factors (S, BP↑, HDL↓)	10	13	15	20	25	28	25	30	33
Evidence of heart disease, angina, a previous heart attack, etc.	20	30	40	25	35	45	30	40	50

* Data are based principally on the Framingham Study.

TABLE 17

APPROXIMATE RISK OF SUFFERING HEART DISEASE FOR 100 MIDDLE-AGED MEN OVER A 10-YEAR PERIOD ACCORDING TO RISK FACTORS*

	AGE 40 SERUM CHOLESTEROL LEVEL (MG/DL)			AGE 50 SERUM CHOLESTEROL LEVEL (MG/DL)			AGE 60 SERUM CHOLESTEROL LEVEL (MG/DL)		
	200	250	290	200	250	290	200	250	290
With no other risk factors	3	5	6	7	9	11	11	14	17
Also is a smoker (S)	6	8	10	11	15	17	17	21	24
Also has high blood pressure	5	7	9	11	14	16	16	20	23
Also has diabetes	5	7	8	9	12	15	15	19	22
With a low HDL (below 35)	7	13	14	13	16	19	19	24	27
With two other risk factors (S and BP↑)	9	12	15	17	21	24	23	28	31
With three other risk factors (S, BP↑, HDL↓)	17	21	24	26	31	35	34	40	43
Evidence of heart disease, angina, a previous heart attack, etc.	30	40	50	35	45	55	40	50	60

* Data are based principally on the Framingham Study. All levels of cholesterol are not included, but you can get an idea of your approximate risk at a low, moderate, and relatively high level.

T A B L E 18

APPROXIMATE RISK OF HEART DISEASE IN WOMEN OVER NEXT 10 YEARS ACCORDING TO RISK FACTORS*

SERUM CHOLESTEROL LEVEL (MG/DL)	Age 40			Age 50			Age 60		
	200	250	290	200	250	290	200	250	290
With no other risk factors					M	M	M	M	M
With one other risk factor: Is a smoker (S)				M	M	M	M	M	M
Has high blood pressure (BP↑)				M	M	M	M	M	M
Has diabetes			M	M	M	M	M	M	M
Has a low HDL (below 35)			M	M	M	M	M	M	M
With two other risk factors (S and BP↑)		M	M	M	M	M	M	M	H
With three other risk factors (S, BP↑, and HDL↓)	M	M	H	H	H	H	H	H	H
Evidence of heart disease, angina, a previous heart attack, etc.	H	H	H	H	H	H	H	H	H

* Data are based principally on the Framingham Study.

□ LOW RISK < 5%   ▨ M­ILD TO MODERATE RISK 5%–20%   ■ H­IGH TO VERY HIGH RISK > 20%

TABLE 19

APPROXIMATE RISK OF HEART DISEASE IN MEN OVER NEXT 10 YEARS ACCORDING TO RISK FACTORS*

SERUM CHOLESTEROL LEVEL (MG/DL)	AGE 40			AGE 50			AGE 60		
	200	250	290	200	250	290	200	250	290
With no other risk factors	□	▒	▒	▒	▒	▒	▒	▒	▒
With one other risk factor: Is a smoker (S)	▒	▒	▒	▒	▒	▒	▒	█	█
Has high blood pressure (BP↑)	▒	▒	▒	▒	▒	▒	▒	█	█
Has diabetes	▒	▒	▒	▒	▒	▒	▒	█	█
Has a low HDL (below 35)	▒	▒	▒	▒	▒	▒	█	█	█
With two other risk factors (S and BP↑)	▒	▒	▒	▒	█	█	█	█	█
With three other risk factors (S, BP↑, and HDL↓)	▒	█	█	█	█	█	█	█	█
Evidence of heart disease, angina, a previous heart attack, etc.	█	█	█	█	█	█	█	█	█

Data are based principally on the Framingham Study.

□ LOW RISK < 5%   ▒ MILD TO MODERATE RISK 5%–20%   █ HIGH TO VERY HIGH RISK > 20%

INDEX

A

Abdominal fat, 13
Achiote paste, 99
Age
  and blood cholesterol levels, 28, 29
  add calorie needs, 13
Aging, and atherosclerosis, 41
Alcohol consumption, and triglycerides, 29
Alcoholic beverages, caloric content of,
    215(t)*
American cuisine, 47
American Heart Association
  Step 1 Diet, 34
  Step 2 Diet, 30, 34
American Place, An, 3, 47
Angel Food Cake, 114–15
Angina, 36
Antioxidant vitamins, 48, 50, 201
Appetizers, 48
  Chilled Oysters with a Cucumber-Mint
    Sauce, 64
  Fish Tartare with Capers, Lemon, and Shal-
    lots, 170
  Grilled Asparagus with Chervil and Hazel-
    nuts, 65
  Grilled Endive with Parsley and Green Pep-
    percorns, 172
  Grilled Soft-Shell Crabs and Sweet Potato
    Salad, 100–01
  Grilled Wild Mushrooms with Parsley and
    Garlic Vinaigrette, 136
  Grilled Young Leeks on Toast, 66–67
  Marinated Sardine Fillets, 137
  Munchkin Pumpkin with Chanterelles and
    Lobster in a Light Curry Broth, 134–35
  Rocket Salad with Baked Ricotta, 98–99
  Spicy Shrimp with Bitter Greens Salad,
    99–100
  Steamed Mussels with Fennel in an Or-
    ange Broth, 171–72
Apple
  and Cranbury Duff, Old-Fashioned,
    152–53
  -Sage Dressing, Roast Chicken with,
    145–47
"Apple-shaped" obesity, 13

---

*(t) = table

B

Apricot Soufflé, 113–14
Artery disease, 5
Arthritis, 11
Artichoke, Grilled New Potato and, Salad,
    96–97
Artichokes
  Chicken Grilled with Citrus, Roasted Gar-
    lic, and, 68–69
  Ragout of Baby, and Stuffed Morel Mush-
    rooms, 63–64
Artichokes, Jerusalem, 124
  Rack of Lamb with, and Mint, 70–71
Arugula, 98
  Sweet Pepper, Eggplant, Tomato, and,
    Sandwich, 88–89
Asparagus
  Grilled, with Chervil and Hazelnuts, 65
  Marinated Seafood Salad with, 95–96
Aspirin, 36
Atherosclerosis, 22, 29, 36, 39–44
  causes of, 41–42
  oxidized LDL in, 48
  risk of, 30
  weight maintenance and, 22
Autumn recipes, 119–53

B

Basil, Fried, Sliced Tomatoes, Grilled Onion,
    and, 86
Bean Soup
  Native, 124–25
  with Wilted Greens and Rosemary Oil,
    176–77
Beans, 66, 161, 162
Beets, Roasted, Endive, and Frisée Salad,
    160
Behavioral changes and atherosclerosis, 41
Beta carotene, 31, 48
Beverages, 201
  alcoholic content of, 215(t)
Black Bean Salad with Grilled Chicken, 30,
    94–95
Black Mission figs, 127
"Binge" eating, 16
Bitter greens, 98
  Spicy Shrimp with, Salad, 99–100

Blood cholesterol, 27, 31
　determinants of amount of, 29–30
Blood cholesterol levels
　and atherosclerosis, 42
　classification of, 28–29, 28(t)
　medications reducing, 35–36
　reducing, 34–35
　reducing by exercise, 33
Blood cholesterol levels, elevated
　and atherosclerosis, 41
　and heart disease risk, 34
　and personal risk, 30
Blood clotting, 10, 29, 36, 49, 50
Blood Oranges, Compote of Tangerines and, 53
Blood pressure, 20, 35
　diet and, 5
　normal, 42
　see also High blood pressure
Blood pressure categories, 43(t)
Blueberries, 82
Body mass index (BMI), 11, 12
Body weight, according to height and BMI, 12
Bourbon Glaze, 75
Bread, 211, 212
Breakfast, 20, 47, 48
　Apple and Pineapple Muffins, 122
　Banana Pancakes, 157
　Buckwheat Crepes with Fruit Compote, 123–24
　Compote of Tangerines and Blood Oranges, 53
　Fresh Herb and Spinach Omelet, 55
　Millet Muffins with Fresh Corn, 81
　Pear, Parsnip, and Potato Pancakes, 158–59
　Ragout of Citrus with Maple Sugar Crisps, 54
　Summer Berry and Maple Pancakes, 82–83
　Summer Vegetable Frittata, 84–85
　Sweet Corn Porridge with Dried Fruits, 159
　in Two-Week Menu Plan, 201
　Warm Apple and Blueberry Compote with Granola and Yogurt, 121
Broccoli, Garlic, Pasta with Grilled Salmon and, 74
Broiling, 49

C

Cake(s)
　Angel Food Cake, 114–15
　Chocolate Cherry Fudge Cake, 76–77
　Lemon Angel Food Chiffon, 115–16, 211
Calamari, White Bean, and Red Lentil Ragout, 161–62
Calcium, 31
Calorie intake, 19, 20, 23
　budgeting, 4, 11
　reduction of, 17, 212
　and weight loss, 9, 13–14, 22, 212
Calorie levels, figuring fat budget by, 18(t)
Calorie needs, age and, 13
Calorie Targets for Losing Weight, 14, 16, 211
Calories
　in alcoholic and carbonated beverages, 215(t)
　burned in exercise, 15(t), 35
　from carbohydrates, 19
　in meat, 19(t)
　percent from fat, 17, 18, 30, 33, 34
　in poultry, 20(t)
　in recipes (this volume), 49, 210
　in Two-Week Menu Plan, 201, 202, 204, 205, 206
　for weight maintenance, 211(t)
Cancer, 11, 42
Carbohydrates, 17
　calories from, 19
Carbon monoxide, 41–42
Carbonated beverages, caloric content of, 215(t)
Cardiology, 3
Celeriac, Braised Veal Shanks with, and Mustard, 6, 18, 184–85
Celery Root
　Purée, Braised Duck Legs with, 178–79
　Smoked Fish and, Salad, 9, 164
Chanterelle, Roasted Corn and, Salad with Autumn Greens, 125–26
Chanterelles, 110
　Baked, with Garlic Toasts, 128–29
　Munchkin Pumpkin with, and Lobster in a Light Curry Broth, 134–35
Cheese, 5, 31
Chefs (this volume), 45–50

Chez Panisse, 3, 47, 48
Chez Panisse Menu Cookbook (Waters), 3
Chicken, 18
    Braised Breast of, Smothered with White
      Beans and Greens, 175–76
    Breast of Pheasant or, with Pumpkin and
      Cranberries, 141–42
    Grilled, Black Bean Salad with, 30, 94–95
    Grilled, Forest Mushrooms, and Red
      Onion Pasta, 73
    Grilled Breast of, with Sweet Corn and
      Wild Mushroom Salsa, 110–11
    Grilled with Citrus, Roasted Garlic, and Ar-
      tichokes, 68–69
    Roast, with Apple-Sage Dressing, 5,
      145–47
    Roast, with Roasted Whole Garlic, 108–09
    Spicy Grilled, with Apples and Chiles,
      150–51
Chicken breasts, 50
Chicken Broth, 193
Chicken Salad
    Provençal, 130–31
    Warm, with Walnut Sherry Vinaigrette,
      168–69
Children, testing for cholesterol, 33–34
Chili, Vegetable Black Bean, 43, 162–63
Chipotle chiles, 112
Chocolate Brownies, Low-Fat, 78
Chocolate Cherry Fudge Cake, 76–77
Cholesterol, 4, 5
    controlling, 31–33
    HDL ratio, 28, 33
    measuring, 28–29
    myths and facts, 25–37
    testing for, 33–34
    in Two-Week Menu Plan, 201, 202, 204,
      205, 206, 207, 208, 209
    what it is, 27
    see also Blood cholesterol; Dietary choles-
      terol; High-density lipoproteins (HDLs);
      Low-density lipoproteins (LDLs)
Cholesterol content of foods, 32(t), 33(t)
    in recipes (this volume), 49, 210
Cholesterol intake, 19, 22, 23, 30, 33, 34
    budgeting, 4
    recipes (this volume) and, 5

Cholesterol levels
    control of, 3
    diet and, 5, 31, 34, 37
    elevated, 13, 27
    exercise and, 35, 37
    and heart attack risk, 10
    lowering, 34–35, 36
    medications to lower, 5, 37
    personal risk for heart disease based on,
      219–22
    and risk, 34
Cholestyramine, 37
Chutney, Tomatillo, Chile-Rubbed Tuna
    with, 112
Cilantro, 64
Citrus, Ragout of, with Maple Sugar Crisps,
    54
Clams, Thyme, and Garlic, Pasta with,
    139
Clinical condition, LDL levels and, 29(t)
Coconut oil, 10
Coffee cart, 213
Colestipol, 37
Common sense, and weight loss, 17–20
Compote
    Buckwheat Crepes with Fruit, 123–24
    of Tangerines and Blood Oranges, 53
    Warm Apple and Blueberry, with Granola
      and Yogurt, 121
    of White Peaches and Nectarines, 113
Cooking for All Seasons (Schmidt), 3
Cooking methods, 49, 50
Cooking styles(s), 48
Corn
    Fresh, Millet Muffins with, 81
    Roasted, and Chanterelle Salad with Au-
      tumn Greens, 125–26
Corn oil, 10
Corn Porridge, Sweet, with Dried Fruits,
    159
Coronary arteries, 41
Couscous, Spicy, Steamed Mussels with Saf-
    fron and, 182–83
Cranberries, Breast of Pheasant or Chicken
    with Pumpkin and, 141–42
Cranberry and Orange Soufflé, 186–87
Crayfish, 62

Crepes, Buckwheat, with Fruit Compote, 123–24
Cucumber-Mint Sauce, Chilled Oysters with, 64

D

Daily requirements, 23
Dairy products, 20, 27, 29, 30, 31
Dessert, 48, 211, 212
  Angel Food Cake, 114–15
  Apricot Soufflé, 113–14
  Baked Figs in Red Wine, 153
  Baked Pear with Wildflower Honey, Wine, and Vanilla, 151–52
  Baked Pumpkin and Walnut Pudding, 189
  Chocolate Cherry Fudge Cake, 76–77
  Compote of White Peaches and Nectarines, 113
  Cranberry and Orange Soufflé, 186–87
  Lemon Angel Food Chiffon, 115–16
  Low-Fat Chocolate Brownies, 78
  Nectarine and Blackberry Crisp, 117
  Old-Fashioned Apple and Cranberry Duff, 152–53
  Pears Poached in Marsala, 188
  Strawberry Granita, 77
Diabetes, 5, 16, 29
  and atherosclerosis, 41
  obesity and, 11, 13
  risk factor, 219
Diastolic blood pressure, 42
Diet
  and atherosclerosis, 41
  balanced, 18–19
  and blood pressure/cholesterol levels, 5
  changing, 4–5
  and cholesterol levels, 5, 31, 34, 37
  and high blood pressure, 35–36
  low-fat, low-cholesterol, 4–5, 18, 42
Dietary cholesterol, 27
  controlling intake of, 31–33
Dietary fat, 5, 9, 47
  and heart attack risk, 27
Diets, dieting, 4, 5, 9
  low-sodium, 43
  "quick fix," 14–16
  vegetarian, 4, 35

Disease(s), obesity and, 11
Dinner, 20, 47, 48
  Baked Salmon, 107
  Baked Salmon with Watercress Sauce, 71
  Barbecued Salmon with Roasted Pepper, Sweet Onion, and Caper Salsa, 109–10
  Bean Soup with Wilted Greens and Rosemary Oil, 176–77
  Braised Breast of Chicken Smothered with White Beans and Greens, 175–76
  Braised Duck Legs with Celery Root Purée, 178–79
  Braised Mahimahi with Fresh Succotash, 105
  Braised Veal Shanks with Celeriac and Mustard, 184–85
  Breast of Pheasant or Chicken with Pumpkin and Cranberries, 141–42
  Chicken Grilled with Citrus, Roasted Garlic, and Artichokes, 68–69
  Chile-Rubbed Tuna with Tomatillo Chutney, 112
  Duck with Dried Cherries and Sage, Mashed Parsnips and Potatoes, 142–43
  Game Hens with Country Ham and Greens Stuffing and Bourbon Glaze, 75–76
  Grilled Breast of Chicken with Sweet Corn and Wild Mushroom Salsa, 110–11
  Grilled Chicken, Forest Mushrooms, and Red Onion Pasta, 73
  Grilled Salmon with Apples and Juniper, 144–45
  Grilled Steak with Gremolata, 138
  Grilled Veal Chops with Summer Garden Salad, 103
  Halibut, Sweet Pea, and Fines Herbes Stew, 67–68
  Herb-Seared Snapper Fillet with Marinated Cucumber and Tomatoes, 104
  Honey-Glazed Grouper, 173
  Mahamahi with Grapefruit and Ginger, 181–82
  Onion and Roasted Pepper Panade, 140
  Pasta with Clams, Thyme, and Garlic, 139
  Pasta with Grilled Salmon and Garlic Broccoli, 74
  Rack of Lamb with Jerusalem Artichokes and Mint, 70–71

in restaurant(s), 212
Roast Chicken with Apple-Sage Dressing, 145–46
Roast Chicken with Roasted Whole Garlic, 108–09
Roast Leg of Lamb with Exotic Spices and Yogurt Sauce, 180
Seared Fillets of Pork with Chili Spices and Maple-Whipped Sweet Potatoes, 174–75
Spicy Grilled Chicken with Apples and Chiles, 150–51
Spring Turnip Soup, 72
Steamed Mussels with Saffron and Spicy Couscous, 182–83
Summer Minestrone, 106
Swordfish with Charred Tomato Vinaigrette, 101–02
Swordfish with Coriander and Chives, 185–86
in Two-Week Menu Plan, 201
Venison Pot Roast with Root Vegetables and Parsnip Whipped Potatoes, 148–49
Dressings
    Citrus, 127
    Lemon-Pepper, 57–58
    Duck Legs, Braised, with Celery Root Purée, 178–79
Duck with Dried Cherries and Sage, Mashed Parsnips, and Potatoes, 142–43
Duff, Old-Fashioned Apple and Cranberry, 152–53

E

Eating
    healthy, 3, 6
    intelligent, 5
    in restaurants, 212
Eating habits, 34
    changing, 19–20, 22
Egg Beaters, 31
Eggs, 5, 27, 29, 31
Elderly (the), 34
    and atherosclerosis, 41
Endive
    Apple, and Walnut Salad, 129–30
    Grilled, with Parsley and Green Peppercorns, 172

Roasted Beets, and Frisée Salad, 160
Endothelium, 42
Estrogen, 33
Estrogen replacement therapy, 36
Exercise, 34
    and blood cholesterol levels, 33
    and blood pressure, 42
    calories burned in, 15(t), 35
    and cholesterol levels, 35, 37
    and high blood pressure, 35–36, 44
    and weight loss, 9, 13, 14
Exercise programs, 4

F

Family history
    of heart disease, 33, 34, 41
    of hypertension, 43
    of obesity, 11, 13
Fast foods, 212
Fat
    in meat, 19(t)
    in poultry, 20(t)
    see also Dietary fat; Saturated fat
Fat budget
    and desserts, 76, 78
    figuring, by calorie levels, 18(t)
Fat-budget diet, 33
Fat budgeting, 3, 4, 5, 9, 17–18, 20–22, 48, 49
    and Two-Week Menu Plan, 201, 202, 203, 205, 209
Fat calories, 5, 30
    in Two-Week Menu Plan, 201, 202, 203, 204, 205, 206, 207, 208, 209
    for weight maintenance, 211(t)
Fat cells, 12, 13
Fat content of foods, 4, 27, 32(t), 33(t)
    in recipes (this volume), 49, 210
Fat distribution, and risk of heart disease, 13
Fat intake, 5, 10, 20–22, 23, 33
    and cholesterol levels, 34
    control of, 3
    how to figure, 17
    monitoring, 17
    percent of calorie intake, 9
    recipes (this volume), 5
Fava beans, 66
FDA regulations, 27

Fennel, 130
Fiber, 31, 201
    sources of, 214(t)
Fiber content, 49–50
Figs, Baked, in Red Wine, 153
Fish, 18, 29, 30, 31, 33, 50
    Baked Salmon, 107
    Baked Salmon with Watercress Sauce, 71
    Barbequed Salmon with Roasted Pepper, Sweet Onion, and Caper Salsa, 109–10
    Braised Mahimahi with Fresh Succotash, 105
    Fish Tartare with Capers, Lemon, and Shallots, 170
    Grilled Salmon with Apples and Juniper, 144–45
    Halibut, Sweet Pea, and Fines Herbes Stew, 67–68
    Herb-Seared Snapper Fillet with Marinated Cucumber and Tomatoes, 104
    Honey-Glazed Grouper, 173
    Mahimahi with Grapefruit and Ginger, 181–82
    Marinated Sardine Fillets, 137
    Pasta with Grilled Salmon and Garlic Broccoli, 74
    Smoked Fish and Celery Root Salad, 9, 164
    Swordfish with Coriander and Chives, 185–86
Fish Broth, 195
Fish fillets, 50, 58
Fish oils, 50
Fish Tartare with Capers, Lemon, and Shallots, 170
Flavor, 47, 49
Focaccia Buns, Garlic and Herb, 196
Food labeling, misleading, 27
Foods
    from animals, 27
    cholesterol content of, 32(t), 33(t)
    low-fat, low-cholesterol, 47
    see also Fat content of foods
Forgione, Larry, 3, 5, 17, 27, 30, 47, 48, 49, 201, 211
Framingham, Mass., study, 27
Frisée, Roasted Beets, Endive, and, Salad, 160
Fruit Compote
    Buckwheat Crepes with, 123–24

Compote of Tangerines and Blood Oranges, 53
Compote of White Peaches and Nectarines, 113
Warm Apple and Blueberry Compote with Granola and Yogurt, 121
Fruits, 20, 27, 31, 48, 50

G

Gallstones, 16
Game Hens with Country Ham and Greens Stuffing and Bourbon Glaze, 75–76
Garlic, 49
    Roasted, Chicken Grilled with Citrus, and Artichokes, 68–69
    Roasted Whole, Roast Chicken with, 108–09
Garlic Toasts, Baked Chanterelles with, 128–29
Gout, 11, 36
Grains, 20, 27, 47
Granola, 121
Grapefruit, 53, 54
Green peppercorns, 172
Gremolata, Grilled Steak with, 6, 18, 138
Grilling, 49
Grouper, Honey-Glazed, 173

H

Halibut
    Sweet Pea, and Fines Herbes Stew, 67–68
    Fillets, Baked, with Tomatoes, Capers, and Fresh Herbs, 58
Hardening of the arteries, *see* Atherosclerosis
Heart attack(s), 5, 22, 36, 41, 44
    blood cholesterol levels and, 35
    obesity and, 11
Heart attack risk, 49
    cholesterol levels and, 10, 27
    exercise and, 35
    obesity and, 13
    reducing, 48
Heart attack risk factors, 3, 4, 5, 35
    diet and, 9
Heart disease, 20, 35, 39–44

blood cholesterol levels and, 28
facts and myths about, 3
family history of, 33, 34, 41
prevention of, 50
and reduction of cholesterol levels, 36
and saturated fat intake, 30
Heart disease risk, 30–31, 33
blood cholesterol levels and, 34
eating for reduction of, 17
elevated cholesterol levels and, 27
fat distribution and, 13
for men, 219, 220(t), 222(t)
personal, based on cholesterol levels,
   219–22
smoking and, 42
triglycerides and, 29
for women, 220(t), 221(t)
Heart disease risk factors, 44
high blood pressure, 42
overweight, 9
Heart failure, 44
Herbs, 20, 48
Heredity
and atherosclerosis, 41
see also Family history
High blood pressure, 16, 30, 35–36, 42
and atherosclerosis, 41, 42
causes of, 43–44
obesity and, 11
as risk factor, 219
treatment for, 43–44
High-density lipoprotein levels, 34
exercise and, 33, 35
in women, 219
High-density lipoproteins (HDLs), 10, 28,
   36, 42
Hydrogenated oils, 10
Hydrogenation, 10
Hypertension, *see* High blood pressure

I

Ideal weight, 14
calories and total fat calories for, 211(t)
calculating, 11
maintaining, 22
Illness, diet-related, 4
Insulin metabolism, 13

J

Jicama, Pineapple, and Watercress Salad, 56
Junk foods, 20

K

Kidney disease, 43, 44

L

Lamb
Rack of, with Jerusalem Artichokes and
   Mint, 70–71
Roast Leg of, with Exotic Spices and Yo-
   gurt Sauce, 180
Leeks, Grilled Young, on Toast, 66–67
Lemon Angel Food Chiffon, 115–16, 211
Lemon-Pepper Dressing, 57–58
Lentils, 161
Life expectancy, 30
Lipo (fat) proteins, 10, 28
Liquid diets, 14, 15, 16
Liver (organ), 13, 36
receptors in, 30, 31
Lobster
Munchkin Pumpkin with Chanterelles and,
   in a Light Curry Broth, 134–35
and Quinoa Risotto, 133–34
Lovastatin (Mevacor), 36
Low-density lipoprotein levels, 29, 35, 36
and clinical condition, 29(t)
Low-density lipoproteins (LDLs), 10, 28, 31,
   42, 50
oxidized, 48
Lower Your Blood Pressure and Live Longer
   (Moser), 42
Lunch, 20, 47, 48
in restaurant, 212
in Two-Week Menu Plan, 201
Lunch and salads
Baked Chanterelles with Garlic Toasts,
   128–29

Lunch and salads (*cont.*)

Baked Halibut Fillets with Tomatoes, Capers, and Fresh Herbs, 58

Black Bean Salad with Grilled Chicken, 94–95

Calamari, White Bean, and Red Lentil Ragout, 161–62

Endive, Apple, and Walnut Salad, 129–30

Grilled New Potato and Artichoke Salad, 96–97

Grilled Vegetable Pasta, 91

Jicama, Pineapple, and Watercress Salad, 56

Little Multicolored Pepper Pizzas, 92–93

Lobster and Quinoa Risotto, 133–34

Marinated Seafood Salad with Asparagus, 95–96

Native Bean Soup, 124–25

Pasta with Bitter Spring Greens, 60

Pasta with Mushrooms, Fennel, and Thyme, 166–67

Poached Oysters and Shrimp with Lemon-Pepper Dressing, 57

Pork Chops with Mustard and Rosemary, 131

Prosciutto with a Roasted Beet and Fig Salad and a Citrus Dressing, 127

Provençal Chicken Salad, 130–31

Radicchio, Watercress, Radish, and Walnut Salad, 61

Ragout of Baby Artichokes and Stuffed Morel Mushrooms, 63–64

Roasted Beets, Endive, and Frisée Salad, 160

Roasted Corn and Chanterelle Salad with Autumn Greens, 125–26

Sea Scallops, Red Peppers, and Marjoram Angel Hair Pasta, 87–88

Seared Sea Scallops with Cranberries and Hickory Nuts, 169–70

Shrimp and Sorrel Risotto, 62–63

Sliced Tomatoes, Grilled Onion, and Fried Basil, 86

Smoked Fish and Celery Root Salad, 164

Spinach, Roasted Pepper, Onion, and Mâche Salad, 132

Spring Greens and Radish Salad, 59

Sweet Pepper, Eggplant, Tomato, and Arugula Sandwich, 88–89

Tomato Confit on Toasted Bread with Pesto, 89–90

Vegetable Black Bean Chili, 162–63

Warm Chicken Salad with Walnut Sherry Vinaigrette, 168–69

Winter Pear, Endive, and Frisée Salad with Crumbled Blue Cheese and Red Wine Vinaigrette, 167–68

Winter Vegetable Salads, 165–66

Lung disease risk, 42

M

Mâche, 132

Mahimahi

Braised, with Fresh Succotash, 105

with Grapefruit and Ginger, 181–82

Maple Sugar Crisps, Ragout of Citrus with, 54

Margarine, 10, 31

Meat(s), 17–18, 27, 30, 31, 48, 50

calories, total fat, and saturated fat in, 19(t)

low-fat, 20

see also Red meat

Medication

with atherosclerosis, 41

for hypertension, 44

to lower cholesterol levels, 5, 35–36, 37

Men

atherosclerosis in, 41

fat distribution, 13

risk of heart disease, 219, 220(t), 222(t)

Menu Plan, Two-Week, 9, 20, 22, 30, 199–215

altering, 201, 209

Minestrone, Summer, 106

Mint, 64

Monosaturated fats, 10

Monounsaturated fat, 31

Morel Mushrooms, Ragout of Baby Artichokes and Stuffed, 63–64

Morels, 166

Muffins

Apple and Pineapple, 122

Millet, with Fresh Corn, 81

Munchkin Pumpkin, 141

with Chanterelles and Lobster in a Light Curry Broth, 134–35

Mushrooms
Forest, Grilled Chicken, and Red Onion Pasta, 73
Grilled Wild, with Parsley and Garlic Vinaigrette, 136
Pasta with, Fennel, and Thyme, 166–67

Mussels
Steamed, with Fennel in an Orange Broth, 27, 171–72
Steamed, with Saffron and Spicy Couscous, 182–83

N

National Heart, Lung and Blood Institute, 3, 29
National Cholesterol Committee, 37
National High Blood Pressure Education Program, 3
Nectarine and Blackberry Crisp, 30, 117
Nectarines, Compote of White Peaches and, 113
New Potato, Grilled, and Artichoke Salad, 96–97
Nicotine, 41, 42
Nicotinic acid (niacin), 36

O

Obesity, 5, 11–13, 14, 29, 30
and atherosclerosis, 41
Obesity gene, 11
Olive oil, 9, 31, 47
Omega-3 oils, 29, 50
Omelet, Fresh Herb and Spinach, 55
Onion, Grilled, Sliced Tomatoes, and Fried Basil, 86
Orange Broth, Steamed Mussels with Fennel in, 27, 171
Ornish Program, The, 4
Osteoarthritis, 11
Overweight, serious/morbid, 16
see also Obesity
Oysters
Chilled, with a Cucumber-Mint Sauce, 64

Poached, and Shrimp with Lemon-Pepper Dressing, 57–58

P

Palm oil, 10
Panade, Onion and Roasted Pepper, 140
Pancakes
Banana, 157
Buckwheat Crepes with Fruit Compote, 123–24
Pear, Parsnip, and Potato, 158–59
Summer Berry and Maple, 82–83
Parsnip Whipped Potatoes, Venison Pot Roast with Root Vegetables and, 148–49
Pasta, 47
with Bitter Spring Greens, 60
with Clams, Thyme, and Garlic, 139
with Grilled Salmon and Garlic Broccoli, 74
Grilled Vegetable, 91
Marjoram Angel Hair, Sea Scallops, Red Peppers, and, 87–88
with Mushrooms, Fennel, and Thyme, 166–67
Red Onion, Grilled Chicken, Forest Mushrooms, and, 73
Pear
Baked, with Wildflower Honey, Wine, and Vanilla, 151–52
Winter, Endive, and Frisée Salad with Crumbled Blue Cheese and Red Wine Vinaigrette, 167–68
"Pear-shaped" obesity, 13
Pears Poached in Marsala, 188
Personal risk, 30–31
Pesto, 197
Tomato Confit on Toasted Bread with, 89–90
Pheasant or Chicken, Breast of, with Pumpkin and Cranberries, 141–42
Pizzas, Little Multicolored Pepper, 92–93
Plaque, 41, 42
Polyunsaturated fats, 10, 50
Pomegranates, 144
Pork, Seared Fillets of, with Chili Spices and Maple-Whipped Sweet Potatoes, 174–75

Pork Chops with Mustard and Rosemary, 131

Portion sizes, 31

Posole, 124

Poultry, 18, 33, 50
    calories, total fat, and saturated fats, 20(t)

Pravastatin (Pravachol), 36

Prevention
    of atherosclerosis, 41
    of heart disease, 3, 50

Processed foods, 20

Prosciutto with a Roasted Beet and Fig Salad and a Citrus Dressing, 127

Protein, 17, 50
    calories from, 19

Psychological problems, obesity and, 11

Pudding, Baked Pumpkin and Walnut, 189

Pumpkin
    Baked, and Walnut Pudding, 189
    Breast of Pheasant or Chicken with, and Cranberries, 141–42

Q

Quinoa Risotto, Lobster and, 133–34

R

Rack of Lamb with Jerusalem Artichokes and Mint, 70–71

Ragout, 70
    of Baby Artichokes and Stuffed Morel Mushrooms, 63–64
    Calamari, White Bean, and Red Lentil, 161–62
    of Citrus with Maple Sugar Crisps, 54

Raspberries, 82

Raspberry Sauce, 115

Rattlesnake Club, The, 3, 47

Recipes (this volume), 3, 4, 5–6, 9, 18, 19–20, 45–50
    arrangement of, 48–49
    calories, fat grams, cholesterol per serving, 27
    ingredients and techniques, 49

integrating with everyday foods, 20–22, 21(t)
    with meat, 17, 18
    nutritional analysis, 49–50
    sodium content, 43
    substitute, 210–11

Recipes, basic, 191–97

Red meat, 5, 29, 31, 47

Restaurant eating, 212

Rice, arborio, 62

Ricotta, Baked, Rocket Salad with, 98–99

Risk factors, 30, 34
    for atherosclerosis, 41–42
    for heart disease, 9, 42, 44
    for stroke, 42

Risotto
    Lobster and Quinoa, 133–34
    Shrimp and Sorrel, 62–63

Rocket Salad with Baked Ricotta, 98–99

S

Safflower oil, 10

Saffron, Steamed Mussels with, and Spicy Couscous, 182–83

St. Thomas' Hospital, London, 4

Salad
    Black Bean, with Grilled Chicken, 30
    Endive, Apple, and Walnut, 129–30
    Grillled New Potato and Artichoke, 96–97
    Grilled Soft-Shell Crabs and Sweet Potato, 100–01
    Jicama, Pineapple, and Watercress, 56
    Marinated Seafood, with Asparagus, 95–96
    Provençal Chicken, 130–31
    Radicchio, Watercress, Radish, and Walnut, 61
    Roasted Beet and Fig and a Citrus Dressing, Prosciutto with, 127
    Roasted Beets, Endive, and Frisée, 160
    Roasted Corn and Chanterelle, with Autumn Greens, 125–26
    Rocket, with Baked Ricotta, 98–99
    Sliced Tomatoes, Grilled Onion, and Fried Basil, 9
    Smoked Fish and Celery Root, 9, 164
    Spicy Shrimp with Bitter Greens, 99–100

Spinach, Roasted Pepper, Onion, and Mâche, 132
Spring Greens and Radish, 59
Summer Garden, Grilled Veal Chops with, 103
Warm Chicken, with Walnut Sherry Vinaigrette, 168–69
Winter Pear, Endive, and Frisée, with Crumbled Blue Cheese and Red Wine Vinaigrette, 167–68
Salads, Winter Vegetable, 165–66
see also Lunch and salads
Salmon
Baked, 107
Baked, with Watercress Sauce, 71
Barbecued, with Roasted Pepper, Sweet Onion, and Caper Salsa, 109–10
Grilled, Pasta with, and Garlic Broccoli, 74
Grilled, with Apples and Juniper, 144–45
Salsa, 84
caper, 109–10
wild mushroom, 111
Salt
content, 50
intake, 43, 44
restriction, 36
sensitivity, 43
Sandwich, Sweet Pepper, Eggplant, Tomato, and Arugula, 88–89
Sardine Fillets, Marinated, 137
Saturated fat, 5, 9, 10, 17, 18, 204, 205, 206, 208 209
in meat, 19(t)
in poultry, 20(t)
percent of calories from, 30, 33, 34
as source of cholesterol, 27
Saturated fat content of foods, 32(t)
in recipes (this volume), 49
Saturated fat intake, 22, 23
and atherosclerosis, 41
and blood cholesterol levels, 31
Sauces
Cucumber-Mint, 64
Raspberry, 115
Watercress, 71
Yogurt, 180
Schmidt, Jimmy, 3, 5, 6, 9, 17, 18, 30, 43, 47–48, 49, 201

Sea Scallops
Red Peppers, and Marjoram Angel Hair Pasta, 87–88
Seared, with Cranberries and Hickory Nuts, 169–70
Seafood Salad, Marinated, with Asparagus, 95–96
Seasonal produce, 3, 6, 47, 48
Sedentary life-style, 41
Self-esteem, obesity and, 11
Sesame oil, 10
Shellfish, 30, 31
Shiitake mushrooms, 73
Shrimp, 31
Poached Oysters and, with Lemon-Pepper Dressing, 57–58
and Sorrel Risotto, 62–63
Spicy, with Bitter Greens Salad, 99–100
Simvastatin (Zocor), 36
Smoking, 5, 22, 30, 35
and atherosclerosis, 41–42
Snapper Fillet, Herb-Seared, with Marinated Cucumber and Tomatoes, 104
Sodium, 20, 43, 50, 210
Soft-Shell Crabs, Grilled, and Sweet Potato Salad, 100–01
Sorrel, 62
Soufflé
Apricot, 113–14
Cranberry and Orange, 186–87
Soup
Bean Soup with Wilted Greens and Rosemary Oil, 176–77
Native Bean Soup, 124–25
Spring Turnip Soup, 72
Summer Minestrone, 106
Soybeans, 10
Spices, 20
Spinach, Roasted Pepper, Onion, and Mâche Salad, 132
Splurging, 5
Spring Greens
Pasta with Bitter, 60
and Radish Salad, 59
Spring recipes, 51–78
Steak, Grilled, with Gremolata, 6, 18, 138
Stew, Halibut, Sweet Pea, and Fines Herbes, 67–68

Stocks, 49, 193–95
Strawberry Granita, 77
Stroke, 41, 44
   risk factors for, 42
Stuffing, Country Ham and Greens, Game
      Hens with, and Bourbon Glaze, 75–76
Succotash, Fresh, Braised Mahimahi with,
      105
Sugar metabolism, 36
Summer recipes, 79–117
Sweet Potato, Grilled Soft-Shell Crabs and,
      Salad, 100–01
Sweet Potatoes, Maple-Whipped, Seared Fil-
      lets of Pork with Chili Spices and,
      174–75
Swordfish
   with Charred Tomato Vinaigrette, 101–02
   with Coriander and Chives, 185–86
Systolic blood pressure, 42

T

Tangerines and Blood Oranges, Compote of,
      53
Thinness, and blood cholesterol, 33
Thyroid gland, 12
Tomatillos, 112
Tomato Confit on Toasted Bread with Pesto,
      89–90
Tomato Vinaigrette, Charred, Swordfish
      with, 101–02
Tomatoes, Sliced, Grilled Onion, and Fried
      Basil, 9, 86
Trans-fatty acids, 10
Triglycerides, 13, 29, 36
Tuna, Chile-Rubbed, with Tomatillo Chut-
      ney, 112
Turnip Soup, Spring, 72

V

Vascular disease, 13, 27
Vascular disease risk, 42
Veal Chops, Grilled, with Summer Garden
      Salad, 103
Veal Shanks, Braised, with Celeriac and Mus-
      tard, 6, 18, 184–85

Vegetable Black Bean Chili, 43, 162–63
Vegetable Broth, 194
Vegetable Frittata, Summer, 84–85
Vegetable Pasta, Grilled, 91
Vegetable Salads, Winter, 165–66
Vegetables, 20, 27, 31, 47, 48, 50
   Venison Pot Roast with Root, and Parsnip
      Whipped Potatoes, 148–49
Vegetarian diet, 4, 35
Venison Pot Roast with Root Vegetables and
      Parsnip Whipped Potatoes, 148–49
Vitamin A, 10, 48, 50
   sources of, 213(t)
Vitamin C, 31, 48, 50
   sources of, 213(t)
Vitamin E, 10, 31, 48, 50
   sources of, 214(t)
Vitamin K, 10
Vitamins, 49
   antioxidant, 48

W

Watercress, 56
Watercress Sauce, Baked Salmon with, 71
Waters, Alice, 3, 5, 6, 9, 17, 18, 47, 48, 49,
      201
Weight, 7–23
   and blood pressure, 42
   see also Obesity; Overweight
Weight control, 11, 17
Weight gain, 13
Weight loss, 3, 9, 13–14
   calorie intake and, 22
   calorie targets for, 14, 16
   common sense and, 17–20
   and high blood pressure, 44
   and reduction of blood cholesterol, 35
   regaining, 14–16
   and triglyceride levels, 29
   and Two-Week Menu Plan, 211–12
Weight Loss Program, examples of how to
      plan, 211, 212
Weight maintenance
   calorie count for, 201
   calorie intake and, 13, 14
   calories and total fat calories for, 211(t)

White Bean, Calamari, and Red Lentil Ra-
    gout, 161–62
White Beans, Braised Breast of Chicken
    Smothered with, and Greens, 175–76
White-coat hypertension, 42
White Peaches and Nectarines, Compote of,
    113
Winter recipes, 155–89
Women
    and cholesterol levels, 34
    fat distribution, 13
    HDL levels, 28, 33
    personal risk, 30
    risk of heart disease, 219, 220(t), 221(t)

Y

Yale University School of Medicine, 3
Yo-yo dieting, 15–16